Poultry Diseases Production and its Management

About the Author

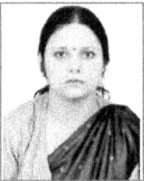

Dr Savita Sharma is an experienced teacher and ardent researcher. She has completed Ph.D in 1998 in CCS. University. Meerut. After selecting in U.P. higher commission She joined the zoology department of D.N. (PG) college. Meerut in 1999.she has 19 years of teaching experience. At present she is continuing the same department in the capacity of Associate Professor. Many students have done PhD. under her supervision in the field of parasitology and Immunology. She is regular member and fellow of various societies and association. She has attended many national and International conferences. She has published several research papers in reputed national and International Journals.

Poultry Diseases Production and its Management

By
Dr. Savita Sharma

2018

Daya Publishing House®
A Division of
Astral International Pvt. Ltd.
New Delhi – 110 002

Published by   :   **Daya Publishing House®**
                            A Division of
                            Astral International Pvt. Ltd.
                            – ISO 9001:2015 Certified Company –
                            4736/23, Ansari Road, Darya Ganj
                            New Delhi-110 002
                            Ph. 011-43549197, 23278134
                            E-mail: info@astralint.com
                            Website: www.astralint.com

Digitally Printed at   :   **Replika Press Pvt. Ltd.**

Preface

Poultry Industry is now becoming one of the largest industry in world. India is also fourth largest producer of egg in the world. The per capita availability of egg & broiler meat is for below the ICMR recommended level of 180 egg and 11 kg meat per annum. The annual contribution of poultry section to the gross national product is about Rs. 7810 crores. Disease in the poultry are major constraints to achieve desired profits. Birds have been threatened by number of infections diseases and nutritional diseases for quiet a long time. Diagnosis at an early stages of the onset of the disease has tremendous implication on successful therapy and implementation of effective control programme. This book has been written to provide a comprehensive picture of different viral, bacterial fungal, parasitic nutritional and metabolic disease this book is very much informative for the students teachers and researches adjoining directly or indirectly with the poultry industry. It contain the information in very simple & understandable manner. Many universities professional colleges and U.P. Board and its intermediate level have introduced vocational courses to supper their financial crunch through self payment and also to encourage educated unemployment youth to take up profession on self employment. Many chapters in this book provide knowledge regarding the maintenance & management of chicks. The authors is confident that this book prove to be most useful to all its reader.

This book is dedicated to my mother who gave me inspiration to do better & beneficial to others in life. The author owes a great deal to her husband in every aspects of life & encourage me to write such type of book. I am also thankful to my son Vidit , Varchasv & my mother in law for their patience & love. I am also thankful to my students Resha for editing the manuscript.

Lastly the author will appreciate receiving comments on quality of book and error if any for further improvement of the book.

Dr. Savita Sharma

drsavitadncollege@gmail.com

Contents

1
POULTRY INDUSTRY IN INDIA

The scientific poultry keeping in India was first initiated and advocated by Christian missionaries. They introduced small flocks of improved breeds from their countries. The performance of these birds were certainly better than desi-fowls and this attracted the attention of Government officials to introduce several model poultry farms in various parts of the country. It happened more so during the World War-II, when army authorities started setting up number of farms with improved birds of egg type to meet the egg demand of defence personnel. This helped to a great deal in popularising poultry farming in the surrounding areas.

A modest beginning towards commercial poultry farming was made during Ist Five Year Plan (1951-55) in which Rs. 2.5 crore was spent on poultry development. Thirty-three extension centres were established for supply of improved breeds of chickens to interested farmers. During 2nd Five Year Plan (1956-60) projects were initiated to encourage both back-yard poultry farming in rural areas and the commercial poultry farming in urban areas. Five regional poultry breeding farms were established to acclimatize the genetically superior stocks imported from foreign countries. As a result of these, poultry feed and equipment industries started developing. A favourable ground thus was prepared to launch a bigger poultry programme during the 3rd Five-Year Plan. Approximately Rs. 2.8 crore was spent during the 2nd Five-Year Plan.

During 3rd Five-Year-Plan, Rs. 8 crore was allotted for poultry programmes but only Rs. 4.5 crore was spent. Other national and international agencies like U.S.A.I.D. (united States Agency for International Developments), Applied Nutrition Programme, F.F.H.C. (Freedom from Hunger Compaign), U.N.D.P. (United Nation Development Programme) came in long way to boost up the poultry development programmes in India. As a result, four franchise hatcheries with foreign collaboration were set up. About 10,000 pure line chicks were imported from Australia. Large scale poultry processing plants were set up in Poona and Chandigarh. All these led to rapid increase in number of commercial poultry farms with improved fowl stock. During the 4th Five-Year Plan, major emphasis was laid on the expansion of poultry marketing facilities. Further the Government of India permitted private sector to establish commercial hatcheries during this Plan.

Agricultural Universities also played a great role by providing well trained personnel for poultry extension and research work during this period. Many universities have created a full fledged department of poultry science. These universities are busy in solving many practical problems of the industry through research. Farmers training is also one of the basic responsibilities of these departments.

The main task during 5th five-Year-Plan was to improve marketing facilities in order to raise the egg production from 7740 million eggs to 11,580 million eggs through commercial poultry farms.

The overall achievement of last 20 years of poultry development in India can be visualized from table 1.1.

Table 1.1: Change in population of laying hens and egg production in India after independence

Year	Laying hens (Millions)	Egg (Millions)	Per capita egg consumption
1961	35	2,520	5.7
1966	39	4,800	10.0
1971	53	6,040	11.0
1976	79	9,290	15.1
1977	82	9,810	16.5
1979	97	12,420	16.6
1981	102	14,280	17.8
1985	140	14,910	18.1
2000	179	15,201	18,9
2004	200	17,120	19.2
2010	250	18,430	19.8
2014	290	18,980	20.2

* State Statistical abstracts.

India with a total of 12,420 million eggs occupies 10th position in the world and comes after U.S.A., USSR, China, Japan, West Germany, U.K., Italy, France and Brazil. Table 1.1 shows the world and regional egg production and consumption data.

The per capita availability of egg in India is one of the lowest in the world. It comes to only about 16 eggs per person per year as compared to 410 eggs in Israel and 200 to 300 eggs per head per year in most of the developed countries.

According to the Nutritional Advisory Committee of I.C.M.R., average Indian diet should consist of among other things half an egg per person per day. On this basis, total requirement for egg in India is over 100,000 millions. Considering that only one-half of the population is potential consumer of egg, we need 50,000 million eggs as against the target to produce 14,000 million eggs by the end of 5th Five-Year-Plan. The gap is very wide, and can be bridged by producing 12 to 15 times more eggs than the present level.

Table 1.2: Poultry population in India (in thousand)

States/UTs	Fowl	Duck	Total Poultry*
India	617734	27643	648829
Andhra Pradesh	123036	766	123981
Arunachal Pradesh	1259	90	1348
Assan	20609	8439	29060
Bihar	10755	499	11420
Chhattisgarh	13838	127	14246
Goa	504	1	505
Gujarat	13327	18	13352
Haryana	28619	33	28785
Himachal Pradesh	725	0	810
Jammu & Kashmir	6487	190	6683
Jharkhand	10448	615	11231
karnataka	41845	13	92068
Kerala	14219	995	15686
Madhya Pradesh	7311	59	7384
Maharashtra	64431	39	64756
Manipur	1830	559	2403
Meghalaya	3026	66	3093
Mizoram	1232	7	1239
Nagaland	2991	120	3156
Odisha	19489	594	20600
Punjab	10536	25	10685
Rajasthan	4914	27	4946
Sikkim	157	1	157
Tamil Nadu	126879	1039	128108
Tripura	2895	756	3701
Uttar Pradesh	8460	270	8754
Uttarakhand	2563	25	2602
West Bengal	73626	12160	86210
Andaman & Nicobar Islands	916	54	979
Chandigarh	129	0	129
Dadra & Nagar havelui	169	0	170
Daman & Diu	25	0	26
Delhi	2	0	2
Lakshadweep	137	26	167
Puducherry	345	35	387

Source: 18th Indian Livestock Census 2007

* Besides fowl and duck, total number of poultry also includes other birds like turkey, quail etc. O-Negligible

Duck Industry in India

In contrast to the extra ordinary development in the field of chicken production in India, the duck production continued to remain neglected in the absence of attention from research workers, developmental agencies and private sector. Duck production thus continued to remain in the hands of poor. In India, duck enjoys the next position after chicken as far as their population is concerned. According to the 1972 Livestock Census, the duck population in the country is about 9 millions which is 7 percent of the total poultry population. They produce about 400 million eggs per year making 5 percent of the total egg output of the country. West Bengal ranks first in terms of duck population, followed by Assam, Tamil Nadu, Andhra Pradesh, Bihar, Orissa and Kerala.

Even though duck keeping is confined to limited area of the country, it contributes to about Rs. 4 crores to national economy per year and provides rural employment to about two to three lakhs rural farmers. Any effort to improve the duck industry will have very great impact on the economic status of these farmers and will create ancillary job opportunities to many others.

Turkey Production in India

At present, turkey production does not figure in any significant way on the poultry scene of India. This situation can change with proper research and extension work undertaken in this area. Consumer education is likely to play very important role in improving turkey production. The turkey production is on increase in North America and in Western Europe.

Constraints in Poultry Production in Tropics (ABROAD)

The basis principles of poultry production in the warn climates are similar to those for temperate climates, namely, good feeding, breeding and management. However, there are certain constraints specific to warm climate like feed resources, availability of good quality birds, disease control etc.

Feed Resources

Less than one fifth of total food grains of world is produced in developing countries. It is not even sufficient for the human consumption of the area. This results in a keen competition between man and livestock particularly non-ruminants for food grains. The inadequacy of food-grains becomes the greatest constraint in the development of poultry industry of developing countries. But it is surprising to note that the poultry industry in developing countries has developed with remarkable speed even when they import food grains. It is possible to use only one-fourth food grains and three-fourth agro-by-products in standard poultry feed to produce high quality protein food like meat and eggs.

In West-Asian countries with high per capita income and strong demand for animal protein it may be economically feasible to develop poultry industry on imported food grains. This is happening in Western Europe and Japan which are major importing countries for grains and vegetable oil cakes for animal feed. This import is growing very fast.

The development of unconventional sources so feed like petro-protein, leaf protein and other sources of high protein and energy are quite promising and likely to reduce competition for food from human beings.

Limited feed supply, should not detract the attention from the possibility of developing of poultry production. Rural poultry production is possible with minimum amount of food grains in the feed, utilizing agro industrial waste and by-products. National policies need to be modified to promote poultry production at rural level.

Availability of Quality Birds

Quality birds can be made available either by importing of improved strains from developed countries or by practising selective breeding of local stock. Selective breeding can only be undertaken if the native stock possess a moderate to high genetic potential for improved performance. Examples of such breeding programmes are "Partridge Green-legs" in Poland, various local breeds in Argentina, the "Wagogo" in Tanzania and the "Dokki-4" inEgypt.

The other type of programe to make available the quality stock is importing the improved strains when the local stock is genetically poor. This type of programme is being followed in India. Quality birds were made available to farmers by importing hybrid birds through foreign collaboration. But now efforts are being made to evolve the improved strains of birds suitable for the need of the country through research. This is being done primarily to get rid of foreign dependence for birds as national policy and secondly to evolve the birds suited to the local agro-climatic conditions.

Marketing

Improved marketing methods are pre-requisites for industrialized poultry production. Lack of organised marketing has been a serious bottleneck in poultry development programme in most of the developing countries. The establishment of co-operative societies could be beneficial to both producers and consumers in many countries. In India, National Co-operative Development Corporation (N.C.D.C.) has started organising poultry marketing on this rational basis. The N.C.D.C. will also organise consumer education and marketing intelligence at country basis.

Disease Control

It is now possible to eradicate or keep under control pullorum disease and it may be possible the same thing with Marek's disease. For other diseases such as New-Castle disease, infectious bronchitis, encephalo myelitis and fowl pox, measures have been developed in most countries to keep them under control.

In developing countries, the establishment of diagnostic centres for diseases and ready supply of vaccines are vital. Government should issue regulations to test periodically the breeding flocks and for proper utilization of vaccines.

Poultry industry serves a very important part in converting grains and other products into eggs and poultry meat for the nutritional benefit of mankind. Providing consumers with food products of superior quality as economically as possible and at reasonable cost is the chief responsibility of agriculture. The poultry industry, in its position as a branch of agriculture, has increased in importance during recent years as a supplier of these products.

Food for humans is of plant and animal origin, certain proportions of plant and of animal products being necessary to provide properly balanced diets for all classes of people. Foods of animal origin provide certain nutrients in which many plant products are more or less deficient. Of particular importance in providing well-balanced diets for growing children, housewives, farmers, industrial workers, and those engaged in sedentary occupations are milk, eggs, red meats, and poultry meat of various kinds.

Whereas foods of plant origin, if consumed in sufficient quantity, provide humans with plenty of energy, foods of animal origin have a higher nutritional value because of their supplies of proteins, minerals, and vitamins in addition to the energy they provide. Grains and most other plant products are relatively low in protein; but milk, eggs, and meat of various kinds have a higher level of protein and contain certain amino acids lacking in plant foods. Amino acids are the nutrients comprising the proteins, several amino acids being very important in human nutrition. Foods of animal origin also supply humans with more of certain minerals and vitamins than do foods of plant origin.

Relative Efficiency of Animal Food Production. Since cows, swine, sheep, beef cattle and poultry are the most important food-producing classes of livestock of this country, it is interesting to compare their relative efficiencies in converting feed into food. From the standpoint of proteins, minerals, and vitamins, milk production is the highest in the efficiency of production. Egg production ranks second in efficiency. Pork production considering the relative amount of fat produced, apparently ranks third. Chicken, duck, goose, and turkey meat production rank above beef and lamb production in efficiency, although beef cattle and sheep utilize forage crops to a greater extent than the various classes of poultry mentioned except geese.

Relative Importance of Poultry Production. The gross poultry income as a percentage of the gross farm income during each of the following 3-year periods was:

1916 to 1918	1925 to 1927	1934 to 1936	1943 to 1945
8.43	11.19	11.57	13.25

The gross poultry income as a percentage of the gross income from livestock and livestock products during each of the following 3-year periods was:

1916 to 1918	1925 to 1927	1934 to 1936	1943 to 1945
17.52	20.74	20.18	23.16

For more than a quarter of century, the relative importance of the poultry industry has steadily increased. At least two reasons are responsible: (1) the relative efficiency of poultry in converting feed into food for humans; (2) the fact that poultry production is not only a farm enterprise that uses relatively inexpensive labor and provides considerable quantities of eggs and meat for home use in addition to products sold but also because there has been considerable commercial expansion of the industry. In 1945 there were 4,900,948 farms on which chickens were reported, this number representing 85.6 percent of all farms in the United States.

Relative Importance of Species of Poultry. The various species of poultry that contribute toward the total poultry income include chickens, turkeys, ducks, geese, guineas, pigeons, and others of less significance. The data in Table 1 show that chickens have been responsible for 91 percent of the total annual poultry income.

Table. 1.3: Percentage of total gross poultry income contributed by each branch of the poultry industry in 1939 and 1945

	1939	1945
Gross egg income	48.8	54.1
Gross farm-raised chicken income	42.2a	27.3
Gross broiler income	a	9.6
Gross turkey income.	7.4	7.8
Gross duck, goose, guinea, etc., income	1.6	1.2
Total	**100.0**	**100.0**

* If any broiler income was reported in 1939, it was include with the gross income from farm-raised chickens.

It is because chickens constitute such a relatively important source of the total poultry income obtained by poultry producers that this book is devoted entirely to problems of producing and marketing chickens and chicken eggs. Problems of raising and marketing other species are discussed in "Raising Turkeys, Ducks, Geese, and Game Birds."

Relative Importance of Branches of the Chicken Industry. During 1945 to 1947, the average annual gross income obtained from eggs, farm-raised chickens, and commercial broilers was $2,955,284,000. Eggs contributed 62.5 percent of this income; farm-raised chickens contributed 27.8 percent; commercial broilers contributed 9.7 percent. During 1945 to 1947 the gross income from commercial broilers amounted to about 26 percent of the gross income from farm-raised chickens and commercial broilers.

Egg and Farm Chicken Production

The chicken industry in the United States has attained its present position of great economic importance as a result of steady growth, and 2, except for a decline during the depression period and a stimulus during the Second World War, because of the great demand for eggs and chicken meat.

The trends of increase in human population and egg production in the United States from 1910 to 1948. From 1925 to 1930, a period of relative prosperity, egg production; but from 1930 to 1935, the depression period with relatively low family incomes, egg production decreased both relatively and absolutely in relation to the human population trend. Unless unforeseen factors affected the human population trend, it is apparent that there will be a demand for increased egg production, especially if per capita consumption remains relatively high.

Although chickens are kept on most farms in practically all sections of the United States, the most heavily populated sections are in certain areas of the Northeastern states, throughout the Middle West, and in limited areas in the Pacific Coast states.

Eggs are produced in great numbers on commercial-poultry farms located in the Northeastern and Pacific Coasts states and in some sections of the Middle West States. At the same time, the very large number of general-farm flocks throughout these regions and in Southern states accounts for the major share of the total egg production.

The number of chickens raised each year follows the same general pattern as that for eggs produced, except that in certain localized areas in some of the states commercial-broiler production is highly concentrated, as indicated by the concentration of black dots

The Leading Egg– and Farm-chicken-producing States. Although poultry raising is carried on in all parts of the country, 15 states are responsible for more than one-half of the eggs produced each year and 15 states are responsible for more than one-half of the farm-raised chickens produced each year.

Table 1.4: gives the rank of the first 15 states with respect to egg production, 1942 to 1946, and the rank of the first 15 states with respect to gross egg income, 1942 to 1946.

State	Eggs produced, millions	State	Gross egg income, thousands of dollars
Iowa	4,138	Iowa	108,916
Minnesota	3,584	Minnesota	96,662
Texas	3,211	Pennsylvania	89,798
Missouri	2,825	Texas	85,529
Pennsylvania	2,675	California	76,602
Illinois	2,658	New York	76,145
Ohio	2,588	Ohio	74,712
California	2,282	Missour	72,848
Wisconsin	2,272	Illinois	70,428
New York	2,169	Wisconsin	63,960
Kansas	2,102	Kansas	53,822
Indiana	1,974	Indiana	53,447
Nebraska	1,854	Nebraska	46,867
Michigan	1,579	Michigan	46,003
Oklahoma	1,455	New Jersey	41,720

The 15 states in the left column of Table 1.4 produced over 68 percent of all eggs produced in the country during 1942 to 1946, and the 15 states in the right column were responsible for almost 70 percent of the total gross egg income obtained during 1942 to 1946.

All the states in the left column of Table 2, except Oklahoma, are also in the right column, although some of them occupy different ranks in the two columns. In spite of the fact that Oklahoma's 1942 to 1946 average egg production exceeded that of New Jersey, the average price of eggs in New Jersey was sufficiently higher than the average price of eggs in Oklahoma to give New Jersey instead of Oklahoma fifteenth place in the right column. The same factor explains the changes of status of some states in the left and right columns. For instance, Pennsylvania occupies fifth place in the left column, but the average price of eggs in the state was sufficiently higher than the average price of eggs in Texas and Missouri that Pennsylvania outranked these two states with respect to gross egg income.

Increase in Rate of Lay. Better breeding methods carried on by poultry breeders, more bred-to-lay males and females used in hatchery flocks, an improvement in the average quality of chicks sold by hatcheries to farmers and commercial-egg producers, the feeding of more completely balanced diets, and more efficient laying-flock management have all contributed to an increased rate of lay during recent years. From 1937 to 1947 the increased rate of lay amounted to over 20 eggs, as shown in Fig. 5. Rate of lay was determined each year by dividing the total number of eggs produced during the year by the average number of layers on hand during the year.

Rate of lay was 14 percent higher in 1947 than in 1942 and 43 percent higher than in 1928, although the number of layers on farms at the beginning of each of the three years was practically the same.

Table 3 gives the rank of the first 15 states with respect to the number of farm-raised chickens produced during 1942 to 1946 and the rank of the first 15 states with respect to gross farm-raised chicken income.

The 15 states in the left column of Table 3 were responsible for over 63 percent of the farm-raised chickens produced in the country during 1942 to 1946, and the 15 states in the right column were responsible for over 64 percent of the total gross farm-raised chicken income during 1942 to 1946.

The states listed in Table 3 are the same as those listed in Table 2, except that Oklahoma and New Jersey are listed in Table 2 but not in Table 3 and North Carolina is listed in Table 3 but not in Table 2.

Small Flocks Predominate. The chicken industry of the United States is largely a farm-flock enterprise. Over 50 percent of the eggs and farm-raised chickens produced each year come from flocks of less than 200 layers per flock. Nevertheless, during recent years an important trend has been the decline in the number of farms producing eggs but an increase in egg production. Figure 6 shows that from 1934 to 1944 the number of farms on which eggs were produced declined from over 5.6 million to about 4.75 million, a decrease of 15 percent.

Table 1.5: The 15 leading states in average annual number of farm-raised chickens produced and in gross farm-raised chicken income, respectively, 1942 to 1946

State	Eggs produced, millions	State	Gross egg income, thousands of dollars
Iowa	55,460	Iowa	60,054
Minnesota	43,850	Pennsylvania	47,105
Texas	43,018	Illinois	40,407
Missouri	37,206	Minnesota	39,387
Illinois	37,012	Ohio	38,177
Pennsylvania	36,572	Missouri	34,168
Ohio	31,987	Texas	33,625
Indiana	30,607	Indiana	32,223
Nebraska	30,504	New York	30,343
Kansas	28,688	Nebraska	26,845
California	25,653	Michigan	26,199
Wisconsin	23,144	Kansas	24,193

New York	22,607	Wisconsin	22,748
North Carolina	22,552	California	22,118
Michigan	21,603	North Carolina	21,601

Most of the decrease in number of farms on which eggs were produced occurred in those farms having less than 50 layers pr flock. There was a slight decrease in the number of farms having between 50 and 99 layers per flock. On the other hand, the number of farms with flocks having between 100 and 199 layers per flock increased from 14.1 percent of the total number of farms in 1934 to 17.8 percent of the total number of farms in 1944. Also, the number of farms having more than 200 layers per flock rose from 5.7percent in 1934 to 10.7 percent in 1944.

Between 1934 and 1944, the most significant changes in the size of laying flocks occurred in the Northeastern, Middle Atlantic, and North Central states, the shift in average size of flock being very pronounced. Relatively little change occurred in the size of laying flocks in the Mountain and Pacific states, since, for the most part, egg production was quite highly commercialized by 1934. Moderate shifts to large laying flocks took place in the South Central states, but in the East South Central and West South Central states laying flocks of less than 100 layers per flock are the rule.

In 1934, 57.5 percent of the farms had less than 50 layers per flock, and these smallest sized flocks were responsible for 17.4 percent of the total egg production, whereas in 1944 the number of these farms having less than 50 layers per flock hand decreased to 49.5 percent of all farms reporting egg production and these flocks produced 12.8 percent of the total egg production (se Fig. 7). On the other hand, in 1934, farms with 200 or more layers per flock produced 36.1 percent of the total egg production, whereas in 1944 farms with 200 or more layers per flock produced 47.8 percent of the total egg production, as shown in Fig. 7.

Shifts toward Commercialization. During recent years there has been a definite trend toward increased commercialization of flocks, both with respect to breeding flocks and market-egg-producing flocks. This increase has occurred principally in the same areas where the principal increases in size of farm laying flocks have occurred. There are over 300,000 commercial-poultry farms in the United States at present.

Broiler Production

The commercial-broiler industry as it is known today had its beginnings in the early 1920's, although "out-of-season" or "hothouse" chickens, as they were often called, were produced in limited numbers in the vicinity of Hammonton, N.J. as early as 1880. About 1920, winter and early spring broilers were grown in New Hampshire, and by 1928 the enterprise was quite extensively developed for those times. The world's most intensive commercial-broiler area had its beginnings in 1923 in the Delmarva Peninsula, which embraces the adjoining countries of Delaware, Maryland, and Virginia. By 1927 broilers were produced extensively in Benton County, Ark.

The primary factors involved in the initial development of the broiler industry were the extreme shortage of fresh-killed poultry during the late winter and early spring months and the discovery that feeding diets supplemented with vitamin D to chickens raised at that time prevented rickets.

Table 1.6 gives the rank of the first 15 states with respect to the number of commercial broilers produced during 1942 to 1946, and the rank of the first 15 states with respect to gross broiler income.

The 15 states listed in Table 1.6 were responsible for 82 percent of all the commercial broilers produced in the country during 1942 to 1946, and for almost 87 percent of the total gross commercial-broiler income during 1942 to 1946.

Table 1.6: The 15 leading states in average annual number of broilers produced and in gross broiler income, respectively, 1942, to 1946

State	Broilers produced, thousands	State	Gross broiler income, thousands of dollars
Delaware	58,735	Delaware	$40,800
Maryland	32,604	Maryland	28,828
Virginia	21,720	Virginia	19,624
Georgia	20,591	Georgia	17,024
Arkansas	15,190	Arkansas	12,080
North Carolina	13,630	North Carolina	11,285
Texas	13,127	California	10,513
California	10,790	Texas	7,922
Connecticut	7,716	Connecticut	7,348
Illinois	7,347	West Virginia	6,821
West Virginia	7,098	Illinois	6,497
Indiana	5,895	New York	5,464
New York	5,878	Indiana	5,427
Florida	5,422	Pennsylvania	5,089
Pennsylvania	5,135	Florida	4,865

A factor of major importance in the commercialization of the Delmarva broiler industry was the relative proximity of that area to the New York City and other eastern markets, overnight truckloads of live broilers being delivered to these markets in the early morning hours. Subsequently, poultry-dressing plants were established which made it possible to deliver dressed broilers to these eastern markets still possessing the "fresh-killed" flavor. That in itself proved to be a tremendous asset.

The principal reasons why commercial-broiler production developed so extensively in such areas as the Delmarva Peninsula, Arkansas, and somewhat later in Georgia, Virginia, and other states include the following: (1) relatively mild winters, (2) relatively low house-construction costs, (3) relatively cheap labor, (4) sandy or other suitable types of soil, and (5) the providing of employment for farmers who were normally engaged in truck-crop production or other agricultural enterprises which required but little labor during the winter months.

Factors Affecting Expansion of Industry. There are several factors to account for the remarkable expansion of the broiler industry during the past few years. Many of these factors will affect the future development of the industry.

One of the most obvious factors that has affected the expansion of the broiler industry has been the increase in the human population. This factor will continue to exercise its influence in future developments. Coupled with this factor of increased population is the factor of increased consumer demand for cut-up chicken ready to fry.

Another factor, not so obvious but nevertheless very important, has been the marked increase over the years in average egg production per hen. Relatively fewer chicks have been purchased by farmers each year for laying-flock replacement purposes than would have been purchased if rate of lay had not increased, and thus relatively fewer surplus cockerels have been marketed than would otherwise have been the case. Also, relatively fewer culled hens have been marketed each year as compared with the larger numbers that would have had to have been sold if average egg production per bird had not increased to the extent that it has.

The fact that broiler production provides relatively quick returns on the money invested in the enterprise as compared with many other branches of farming is another reason why so many people have become interested in raising broilers.

A factor that has resulted in greater efficiency of operation during recent years, and thus has tended to expand the industry, has been the construction of wider buildings equipped with central-heating systems, automatically controlled mechanical feeders, and automatically controlled waterers, all of which have meant that many more broilers can be cared for per man than formerly. In addition, these wider houses make possible the use of a manure spreader or truck in cleaning out the house, thus reducing labor requirements for this particular job.

Still another factor that has affected the increased consumer demand for fresh-killed, cut-up chicken ready to fry, and thus has influenced further growth of the broiler industry, has been relatively high level of consumer purchasing power that has prevailed during recent years.

The future development of the commercial-broiler industry will be affected by all these factors and in addition by the future per capita consumption of broilers, which will be influenced by improvement in quality of broilers sold, competition from red meats, and family incomes.

The Hatchery Industry

The commercial development of the hatchery industry had its beginnings in the 1880's, although it was not until the manufacture of mammoth incubators in the 1890's that the hatchery expanded to an appreciable extent. A significant stimulant to the industry occurred when chicks were admitted to the mails on May 15, 1918.

In 1928 about 32 percent of all chicks hatched in the United States were hatched in commercial hatcheries, whereas by 1947 the figure has risen to about 90 percent.

In 1938, there were 10,531 hatcheries with a capacity of 397,376,000 eggs. In 1943, there were 10,112 hatcheries with a capacity of 504,640,000 eggs. In 1948, there were 9,341 hatcheries with a capacity of 551, 847,000 eggs.

Figure 10 shows the effects of the period of economic depression, 1930 to 1935, on the decreased demand for chicks. Beginning about 1936 the continued expansion of the broiler industry led to increased hatchery output, which was greatly accelerated during the Second World War. Also, during the war period, there was greatly increased demand for chicks for laying-flock replacement purposes and for "broiler" chicks.

Table 1.7 gives the rank of the first 20 states with respect to numbers of chicks hatched during 1942 to 1946.

Table 1.7: The 20 leading states in average annual number of chicks hatched, 1942 to 1946

State	Chicks hatched, thousands	State	Chicks hatched, thousands
Missouri	112,695	Kansas	43,792
Illinois	106,266	Virginia	36,785
Indiana	103,687	Delaware	35,927
Iowa	102,190	North Carolina	34,519
Ohio	76,496	Nebraska	34,183
Minnesota	68,066	Michigan	32,138
Pennsylvania	67,776	New Jersey	31,044
California	64,400	Connecticut	29,866
Texas	60,429	Oklahoma	29,694
Maryland	52,216	Georgia	29,305

These 20 states were responsible for over 81 percent of the chicks hatched in the country during 1942 to 1946. The first 10 states in the left column were responsible for 71 percent of the chicks hatched in the country during 1942 to 1946.

Cash Poultry Income

Since 1910 the trends in cash income from eggs and farm-raised chickens show wide fluctuations, s indicated in Fig. 11. The impact of the First World War, the serious economic depression during the early thirties, and the Second World War affected both volume of production and prices, which in turn affected cash farm income. Broiler production, being a relatively recent development, has not experienced the same fluctuations in cash income as the other branches of the chicken industry.

Two factors of major importance in the marked increase in each farm income from eggs, farm-raised chickens, and broilers from 1942 to 1947 have been higher prices and increased per capita consumption of eggs and chicken meat.

During 1945 to 1947, the value of eggs consumed on the producers premises amounted to slightly over 14 percent of the total gross egg income. The value of the farm-raised chickens consumed on the producers premises was over 22 percent of the gross farm-raised chicken income and over 16 percent of the gross income from farm-raised chickens and broilers.

A Valuable Asset

The chicken industry is a valuable asset, since it not only provides consumers with highly nutritious food products but adds several million dollars annually to the income obtained from agriculture. Also, many millions of tons of feed are converted into food products on a relatively efficient basis. On many farms, family labor in caring for the flock is utilized more advantageously than is possible with numerous other enterprises.

The production of eggs and chicken meat provides employment not only for those engaged in the production of these products but also for hatchery operators, feed dealers, manufacturers of incubators, equipment, building materials, egg cases, poultry coops, cars, and trucks, processors of egg and poultry products, and all dealers engaged in the marketing of eggs and poultry from the time they leave the producers premises until they are in the hands of the consumers.

Some conception of the magnitude of the chicken industry may be gained by a glance at the following average annual figures for 1942 to 1946, inclusive:

No. of layers on hand on Jan. 1..................................	477,714,000
No. of layers on hand during the year......................	369,875,000
No. of eggs produced...	54,627,000,000
No. of chicks hatched..	1,412,843,000
No. of farm-raised chickens produced......................	760,024,800
No. of commercial broilers produced.......................	273,148,800
Gross egg income..	$1,578,569,800
Gross farm-raised chicken income............................	775,677,000
Gross commercial-broiler income.............................	239,710,400
Total gross income...	$2,593,957,200

The chicken industry has demonstrated its ability to adjust itself, for the most part, to changing economic conditions and maintain itself as one of the most stable and important branches of agriculture in the United States.

2

DIFFERENT BREEDS OF CHICKEN

The original habitat of the ancestor of modern breeds of chickens is south and central India, the Himalayan Terai, Assam, Burma, Ceylon, and throughout all the countries to the southward, on into Sumatra and Java with its string of lesser islands to the eastward. There are four known species of wild fowl, and they belong to the same genus called "Gallus", meaning a cock.

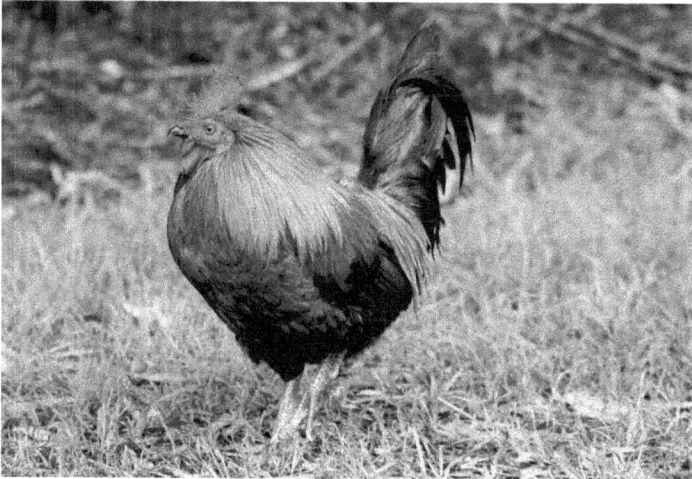

Fig. 2.1

The four species are as follows: (1) Gallus gallus or Gallus bankiva, the Red Junglefowl; (2) Gallus lafayetti, the Ceylon Junglefowl; (3) Gallus sonneratti, the Grey Junglefowl; (4) Gallus varius, the Javan Junglefowl. The Javan Junglefowl differs from the other three species in having a single-median wattle, a smooth-edged comb, truncated neck hackles, and an extra pair of rectrices, or tail feathers.

The general distribution of the four species is as follows: The Red Junglefowl is widely distributed through eastern India, Burma, Siam, and Sumatra; the Ceylon Junglefowl in Ceylon; the Grey Junglefowl in western and southern India; the Javan Junglefowl in Java and adjacent islands.

All four species will cross with one another, and the hybrids are more or less fertile among themselves. Also, from evidence supplied by naturalists and investigators who have made crosses between each of the four wild species and domestic stocks, it appears that all hybrid progeny are fertile, with the possible exception of the female offspring of the cross between the Gallus varius male and domestic females. Apparently, most of the modern-day breeds are descended from these four wild species.

The sport of cockfighting exercised a tremendous influence not only in the domestication of cockfighting exercised a tremendous influence not only in the domestication of wild birds but also in the subsequent distribution of the fowl throughout the world.

In 1873 there took place the first organized effort in the United States to place the poultry-breeding industry upon a stable basis. In that year the American Poultry Association was organized, which had for its object the formulation and adoption of a standard of excellence to be used exclusively by poultry associations in awarding prizes on exhibition poultry. A complete standard was adopted for all the then recognized first "Standard of Perfection" was printed. Since that time, the "Standard", revised periodically, has served as the basis of guidance in breeding operations in developing many breeds and varieties. In many respects, therefore, the standard bred poultry industry served as a foundation for the subsequent development of the industry.

Breeds and Varieties: The Breeds and varieties of chickens are so numerous that a detailed discussion of all the characters they possess is not possible in this book. Moreover, the reader is referred to the "American Standard of Perfection", published by the American Poultry Association, and to the other works listed at the American Poultry Association, and to the other works listed at the end of this chapter.

The breeds are classified largely from the standpoint of their origin, emphasis being placed upon the more important characteristics of economic importance in the more popular breeds and upon the unusual characteristics of those breeds and varieties bred largely for pleasure.

Breed Type: The distinguishing feature whereby one breed of fowls differs from another breeds is in respect to type, although this is rather a confusing situation, in as much as the visible body type is influenced not only by the actual shape of the body but also by the feather contour. In breeding standard bred poultry, the "type" of bird, as determined by feather contour, has been regarded as of greatest importance, so much so that in many cases the actual body type has received minor attention. It is now recognized that "shape makes the breed", shape here indicating very largely feather contour.

Variety Colors: Within each breed of fowls there naturally was a tendency to segregate various color combinations, or, where only one color existed in the original breed, there was a tendency to develop new color patterns. In either case, it was necessary to adhere to the original type or shape characteristic of the breed, and thus it has arisen that varieties of a breed are supposed to be identical in all characteristics except plumage color or, in some cases, in respect to the type of comb, standard weight, color of shanks, and other minor characteristics. There is a large grain of truth in old saying of poultry breeders that "shape makes the breed and color the variety."

The illustrations in the accompanying pages are designed to present the standard type various breeds and should be studied closely. The problem of an adequate color description for the numerous varieties is simplified materially, because there are relatively few standard color patterns. For instance, the color pattern of the Dark Brahma, Silver Penciled Plymouth Rock, and Silver Penciled Wyandotte are almost identical, as is also the case with the color patterns of the Light Brahma, Columbian Plymouth Rock, and Columbian Wyandotte. The plumage pattern and feather markings of the Partridge Cochin are identical with those of the Partridge Plymouth Rock and Partridge Wyandotte. In certain breeds there are silver-laced and golden-laced varieties, in the latter the white of the silver-laced variety being replaced by red and reddish brown. There are black varieties and white ones of many breeds, and there are blue varieties of a few breeds, in each case the color being identical.

The standard weights of representative breeds are given in Table 6, and the type of comb and color of ear lobe, skin, shanks, and egg of these same breeds are given in Table 7.

AMERICAN BREEDS

A number of breeds have been developed in America to meet the marekt demand for a bird with a yellow skin, unfeathered shanks, and adapted to the conditions of the country. With one or two exceptions all American breeds have yellow shanks; except for the Lamona, all have red ear lobes; all lay brown-shelled eggs.

Chickens of relatively small size with black-and-white bars and usually with rose combs were common in many parts of the eastern United States as early as 1750. They were recognized under the breed name of Dominique, but their popularity soon waned.

Plymouth Rock: The Plymouth Rock is rather long bodied, fairly broad, and with fairly prominent breast and good depth of body. The varieties of Plymouth Rock include the Barred, White, Buff, Blue, Columbian, Partridge, and Silver Penciled.

In the development of the *Barred Plymouth Rock*, Dominique breeding stock was used to some extent but the black-and-white barring is much more distinct in the former than in the latter. In the barred Plymouth Rock male the black-and-white bars should be of equal width, whereas in the Barred Plymouth Rock females the white bars should be one-half as wide as the black bars.

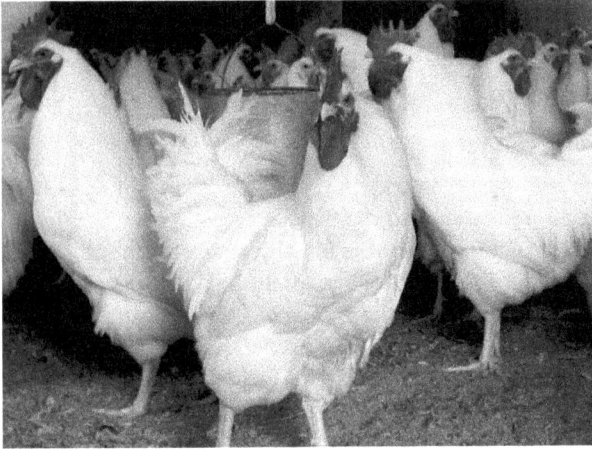

Fig. 2.2

In the *White Plymouth Rock*, the plumage color is pure white throughout and should be free from black ticking, brassiness, and creaminess, as should be the case with all white varieties of other breeds.

The plumage color of the *Buff Plymouth Rock*, as in buff varieties of other breeds, is golden buff in all parts of the surface color, and all sections should be of the same shade. The undercolor is of lighter shade than the surface color.

The Columbian Plymouth Rock was developed from crosses between Light Brahmas and White Plymouth Rocks. Most of the plumage is white, although the hackle feathers of the male and the neck feathers of the female and the tail coverts of both sexes are black, with a distinct white lacing. The tail feathers in both sexes are black. The wings also carry some black on the primary and secondary feathers, which is almost hidden when the wings are folded. The undercolor of all sections in both sexes should be light bluish slate.

The *Silver Penciled Plymouth Rock* owes its feather markings, to a considerable extent, to the Dark Brahma. It has a distinctive color pattern in which the male differs considerably from the female.

The plumage of the male consists of as silvery-white surface color, extending over the wing bows and back, and the hackle and saddle are silvery white, striped with black. The rest of the plumage, including the main tail feathers and sickles, is black. the primaries are black, except for a narrow edging of white on the lower edges of the lower webs, and the secondaries are also black, with some white.

In the female the general surface color is gray, with a distinct, concentric penciling of dark gray on each feather. The neck feathers are silvery white, with a black center showing a slight gray penciling, and the main tail feathers are black, with the two top feathers showing some penciling. In both sexes the unercolor is slate, shading to a lighter color toward the base in the male.

The *Partidge Plymouth Rock*, developed apparently from Partridge Cochins and Brown Leghorns, in color pattern is practically the same as the Silver Penciled Plymouth Rock, except that the white in the Silver Penciled is replaced by red or reddish brown.

The hackle of the male is greenish black with a narrow edging of brilliant red; the plumage in from of the neck is black. The wing bow is brilliant red. The primaries are black, with the lower edges reddish bay, and the secondaries are also black, the outside web of reddish bay with greenish black at the end of each feather. The back has brilliant-red feathers, each with a greenish-black stripe down the middle.

In the female the neck is reddish bay, and the front of the neck and breast are both deep reddish bay, distinctly penciled with black. The wing bows are also deep bay penciled with black. The primaries are black with an edging of deep reddish bay on the outer webs, the inner webs of the secondaries are black, and the outer webs are reddish bay deeply penciled with black. The back is also deep reddish bay penciled with black. The undercolor of all sections of both sexes should be slate. The beak is dark horn shading to yellow at the tip.

The *Blue Plymouth Rock* has plumage of an even shade of blue, each feather being laced with darker blue, and it the male the lacing of the wing bows, hackle, back, saddle, sickle feathers, and tail coverts is very dark. This general description fits other blue breeds and varieties. (See the discussion on the inheritance of blue plumage under Blue Andalusians in the section on Mediterranean breeds.)

Rhode Island Red: The Rhode Island Red has a rather long, rectangular body. This breed was developed from matings of Red Malay game cocks to the common hens of Rhode Island and from matings between rose-comb Brown Leghorns and mottled females.

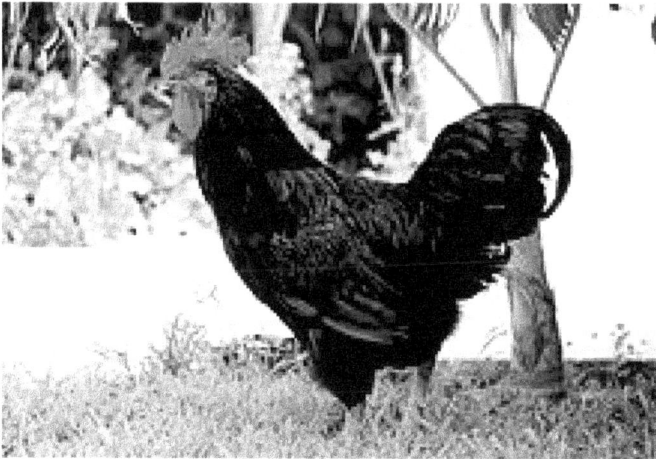

Fig. 2.3

The plumage color of the Rhode Island Red is a rich brownish red which should be as even as possible over the entire surface and throughout all sections, except that the lower webs of the primaries are mostly black; the upper webs of the secondaries are partly black; and the tail coverts, sickle feathers, and main tail feathers are black. In the lower neck feathers of the female there is also a slight ticking of black. The undercolor of all sections in both sexes should be red and free from a dark or slaty appearance, which is known as "smut." The beak is reddish horn, and the shanks and toes are rich yellow or reddish horn.

Rhode Island White: The Rhode Island White, of which the rose comb is the only variety, is identical in size and type with the rose-comb Rhode Island Red and was developed from White Wyandottes, Partridge Cochins, and rose-comb White Leghorns. The plumage should be pure white, free from any tint of brassiness.

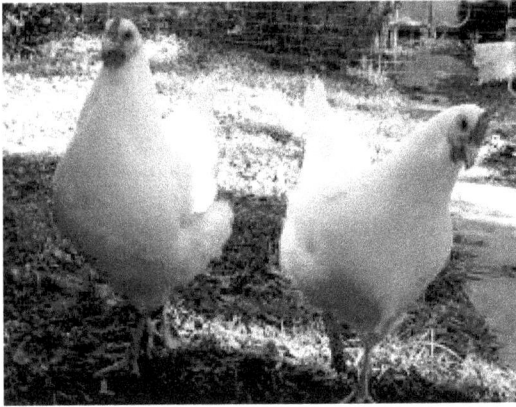

Fig. 2.4

New Hampshire: The New Hampshire breed was developed in New Hampshire from fast-growing, light-colored strains of Rhode Island Reds. The New Hampshire has a single comb. In shape of body the New Hampshire is less rectangular in shape than the Rhode Island Red. In the New Hampshire male the back is brilliant deep chestnut red, and the wing fronts, breast, body, and fluff are medium chestnut red. The saddle is brilliant chestnut red, and the main tail feathers are black, as are the lower webs of the primaries. The neck feathers are brilliant reddish bay.

In the New Hampshire female the neck, wing fronts, primary coverts, back, breast, body, and fluff are medium chestnut red. The lower neck feathers are distinctly tipped with black. The main tail feathers are black, edged with medium chestnut red. In both sexes the undercolor is light salmon.

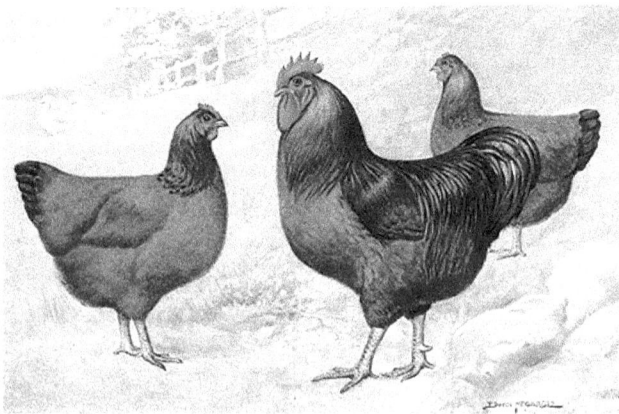

Fig. 2.5

Delawares: The Delawares represent on of the newest members of the American breeds. They were developed from selected progeny secured from crossing Barred Plymouth Rock males and New Hampshire females. The chicks that served as foundation stock of the breed that came to be recognized as Delawares were white in color at hatching time. As adults, they had white plumage except for black-and-white barring in the neck, wing, and tail feathers. Several years of selection and breeding for uniformity in plumage pattern resulted in the recognition of the Delawares as a breed. Rapid growth and fast feathering were given particular emphasis in the selection and breeding program.

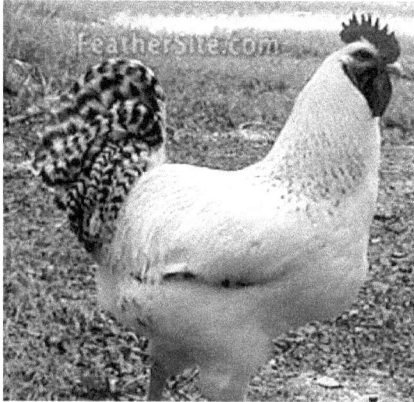

Fig. 2.6

The body is broad and deep, and the back is broad, sloping slightly from the saddle to the tail. The breast is deep and full.

Wyandotte: The body of the Wyandotte is comparatively round, and the general shape and character of feathering give it an appearance of having a rather short back and being low et.

The Silver Laced Wyandotte was the first variety developed, principally from crosses between Buff Cochins and Silver Sebright Bantams and from crosses between Dark Brahmas and Silver Spangled Hamburgs. This variety has a striking color combination which makes it very attractive.

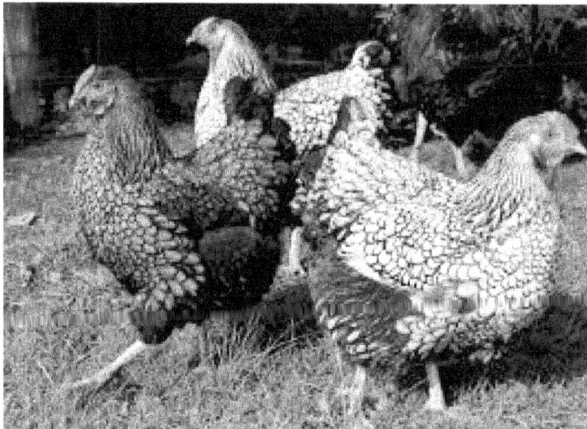

Fig. 2.7

The male has a silvery-white hackle, back, and saddle, the hackle and saddle feathers being striped with black. The feathers of the body and breast are white, laced with a black edge. The primaries are black with the lower edges white; the secondaries are also black with the lower half of the outer webs white and the upper webs edged with white. The main tail feathers are black.

The female has white feathers laced with black over the entire body, except the neck feathers, which are black; there is also some black in the wings. The primaries and secondaries are practically the same as in the male. In both sexes the undercolor is slate. Other varieties of Wyandottes include the White, Buff, Black, Columbian, Golden Laced, Partridge, and Silver Penciled.

Other American breeds include the Jersey White Giant, Jersey Black Gaint, Java, Buckeye, Lamona, Chanticler of Canadian origin, and Cubalaya of Cuban origin.

ASIATIC BREEDS

Of the three Asiatic breeds recognized as standard, the Brahma, Cochin, and Langshan (Fig), only the first two ever gained particular prominence in the American poultry industry. With the development of the American breeds, however, the popularity of the Asiatic breeds was not maintained, and they are now bred to a limited extent only.

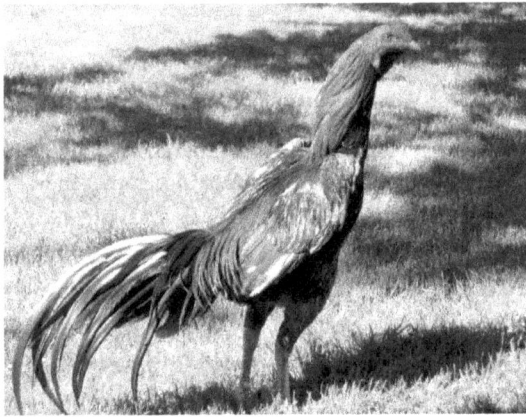

Fig. 2.8

The breeds belonging to the Asiatic class are of distinctive type and have large bodies, feathered shanks, and are usually heavy in bone. All have yellow skin, except the Black Langshan, whose skin is a pinkish white. All have red ear lobes, lay brown-shelled eggs, and are classed as broody.

The three Asiatic breeds include the Brahma, Cochin, and Langshan. There are three varieties of Brahmas: the Buff; the Light, which has the same color pattern as the Columbian Plymouth Rock; and the Dark, which has the same color pattern as the Silver Penciled Plymouth Rock. There are four varieties of Cochins; the Buff, Black, White, and the Partridge, which has the same color pattern as the Partridge Plymouth Rock. The Langshan varieties include the Black and the White.

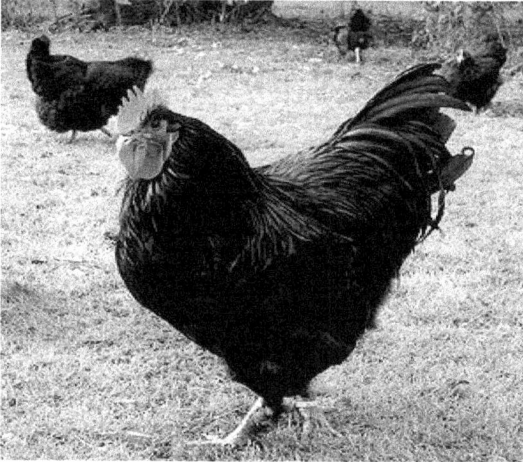

Fig. 2.9

English Breeds

The breeds of English origin described in the "American Standard of Perfection" are, for the most part, utility breeds noted for their excellent fleshing properties. With the exception of the Cornish, all the breeds have white skin and red ear lobes and, except the Dorking and Red Cap, lay brown-shelled eggs. All are classed as broody.

The six English breeds include the Orpington, Australorp, Dorking, Sussex, Red Cap, and white Cornish (Fig.). The Orpingtons are characterized by their size and shape of body, which is long, deep, and well rounded, with a full breast and broad back.

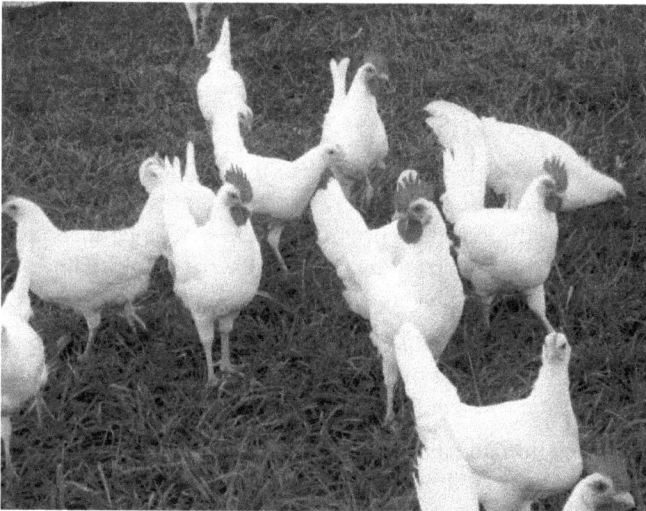

Fig. 2.10

There are four varieties of Orpingtons, the Buff, Blue, Black, and White. The Dorking is a five-toed breed in which the body is long, broad, deep, and low set. There are three varieties of Dorkings, the White, Colored, and Silver Gray. The Australorp (Fig.11) was developed in Australia from the Black Orpington but is more upstanding and less massive in appearance. In the Sussex breed the body is long, broad at the shoulders, and with good dept from front to rear.

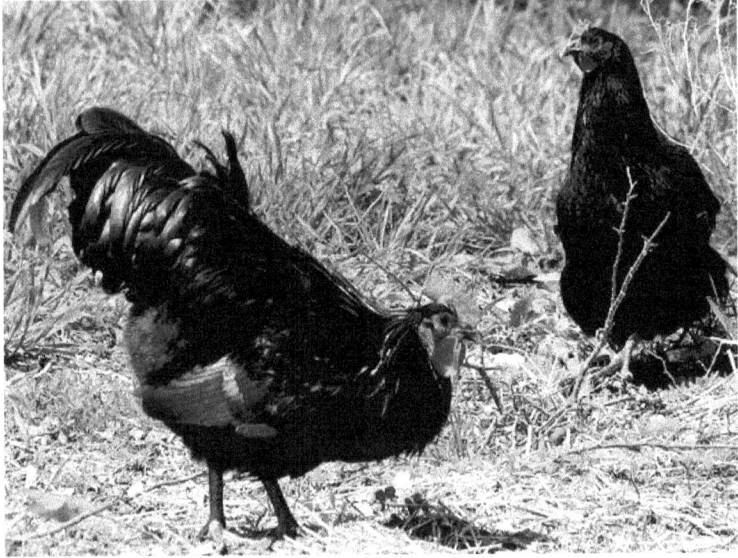

Fig. 2.11

There are three Sussex varieties, the Light, whose color of plumage is quite similar to the Columbian Plymouth Rock, the Red, and Speckled. The Red Cap is a bird of medium size and has a rose comb. The Cornish is noted for its close feathering and compact, heavily meated body, which has a distinctive shape. The breast is very deep and broad, giving the shoulders great width. There are three varieties of Cornish, the Dark, White and White Laced Red.

MEDITERRANEAN BREEDS

The breeds of Italian origin are smaller than the Asiatic breeds, and in America the White Leghorns especially have been bred for egg production rather than for the production of table poultry. The breeds of Spanish origin are somewhat larger than the Leghorns and Anconas. All the Mediterranean breeds have non-feathered shanks, white or creamy-white ear lobes, lay white-shelled eggs, and are relatively non-broody.

Leghorn: The Leghorn is noted for the graceful blending of its different sections and its stylish carriage. All the varieties of Leghorns have yellow beaks, skin, shanks, and toes. There are single-comb and rose-comb varieties.

The single comb in the male should be of medium size and should stand erect, with five regular, deeply serrated points, the back of the comb extending straight out from the back of the head. In the female the front of the first point should stand erect, but the remainder of the comb should droop to one side. The comb in both sexes should be free from wrinkles, "thumbmarks", or folds.

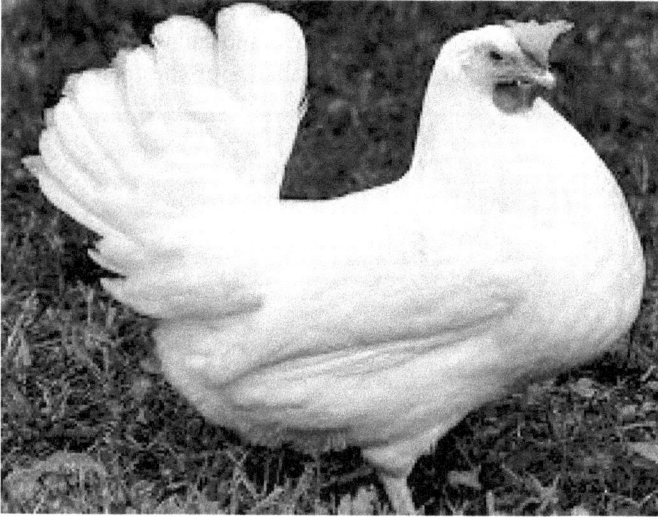

Fig. 2.12

In the rose-comb variety the comb of the male should be of medium size and square in front, well filled and free from hollows, the spike well developed and extending straight back from the head. In the female the comb is small, neat, and in shape is like that of the male.

There are 12 varieties of Leghorns, the Buffs, Blacks, Reds, Silvers, Columbians, and Black-tailed Reds having single combs only, whereas there are single-comb and rose-comb sub-varieties of the Whites, Dark Browns, and Light Browns.

Ancona: The Ancona resembles the Leghorn in type and has black plumage except for certain feathers with a white tip. Over the back and saddle of males, one feather in five is tipped with white; over the back of females, one feather in about two is tipped with white. Over the breast, body, and fluff in both sexes, one feather in about two is tipped with white.

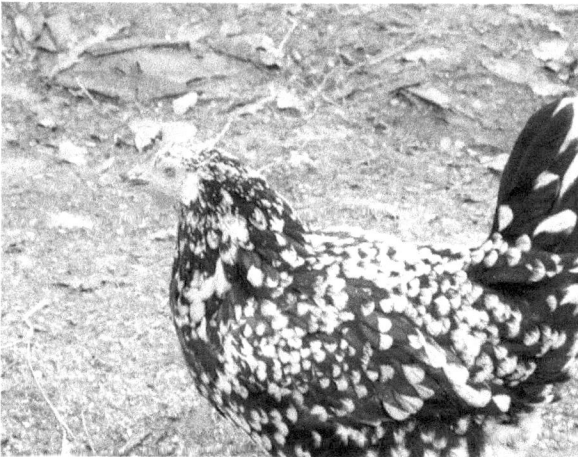

Fig. 2.13

Minorca: The Minorca is the largest of the Mediterranean breeds and is noted for its length of body, downward sloping back, and large comb and wattles. The varieties include: Blacks and Whites, each with single-and rose-comb sub-varieties, and the Single-comb Buff.

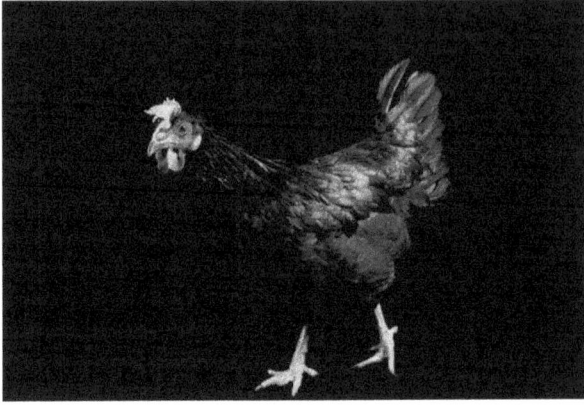

Fig. 2.14

White Faced Black Spanish: This breed has a very extensive white face, the body type being similar to the Minorca.

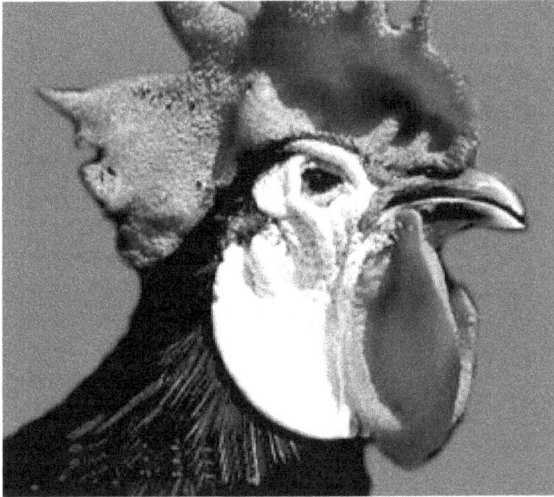

Fig. 2.15

Blue Andalusian: The color of this breed is similar to that of the Blue Plymouth Rock. The Blue Andalusian has not been bred extensively for egg production, but is of interest particularly with respect to the inheritance of its blue plumage.

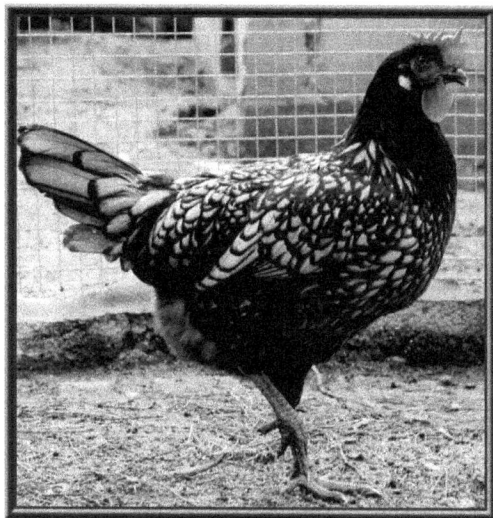

Fig. 2.16

The progeny of Blue Andalusian male and female parents comprise three groups in the following proportions: 1 black to 2 blue to 1 white; splashed with blue. Black males and females mated together produce blacks, and blue-splashed white males and females mated together produce blue-splashed whites. Typical Blue Andalusians result from matings of opposite sexes of blacks and blue-splashed whites, as well as (for one-half of the progeny) when Blue Andalusian males and females are mated together, as explained above.

Buttercup: The two outstanding features of this breed are its cup-shaped comb and the golden ground color of its plumage.

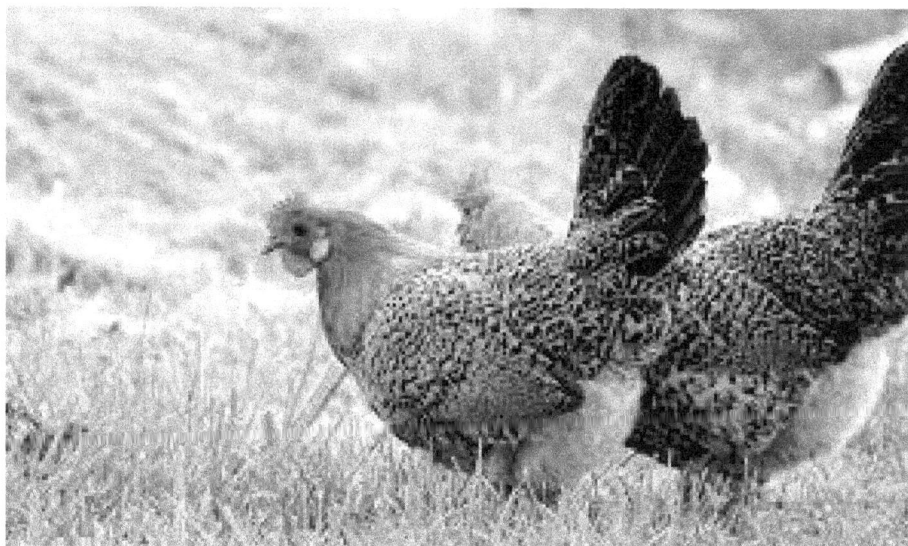

Fig. 2.17

OTHER BREEDS

Among several Continental European breeds, the Houdan, La Fleche, Faverolles, and Crevecoeur are of French origin, but none of them has become popular in the United States. The Campine is of Belgian origin and includes the Silver and Golden varieties. Interest in the Campine lies largely in the fact that the males are hen feathered, the hackle, saddle, and lesser tail feathers being of the same shape as in the female. There are several varieties of the Polish breed, its outstanding feature being a well-developed crest surmounting the head. There are also several varieties of the Hamburg breed, an outstanding character being the upturned spike of its Hamburg breed, an outstanding character being the upturned spike of its rose comb. There are numerous varieties of the Game breed, bred to a limited extent only by fanciers.

Three miscellaneous breeds recognized as standard in America include the Frizzle, with its peculiar development of the feathers which show a tendency to curve outward at their ends; the Silkie, with its blue skin and silky-appearing feather formation; and the Sultan, with its V-shaped comb, a crest, muffs, beard, and vulture hocks.

The Phoenix or Yokohama, of Japanese origin, is interesting because some of the saddle feathers are developed to extreme length, sometimes as long as 20 ft. The Araucana, of South American origin, is of interest because it has a peculiar growth of feathers on each side of the neck, is frequently rumpless, and lays a light-blue-tinted egg. The Creeper is noted for its extremely short legs. There are numerous breeds of bantams, of interest to fanciers only.

DEFECTS AND DISQUALIFICATIONS

Very few birds attain perfection in type, plumage color, and other characters. Imperfections are classed as defects or disqualifications, the latter barring a bird from winning a prize in a poultry show where the "Standard of Perfection" is used as the basis of judging the entries.

Defects include such things as too few or too many points on single combs, color of eyes other than as described for the breed, crooked toes and keels, creaminess in plumage of white varieties, and black feathers in Barred Plymouth Rocks.

Disqualifications include such things as deformed beaks, side spring in single-comb varieties, positive enamel white in the ear lobe of American and Asiatic varieties, and decided bowleggedness or knock-kneedness.

In the selection of breeding stock, disqualifications and defects of major importance should always be kept in mind, especially those that are inherited.

Table 2.1: Standard Weight of Pounds in Some Representative Breeds

Breeda	Cock	Hen	Cockerel	Pullet
Ancona	6	4½	5	4
Australorp	8½	6½	7½	5½
Brahma (Light)	12	9½	10	8
Cornish (Dark)	10	8	8½	6½
Delawares	8½	6½	7½	5½
Jersey Black Giant	13	10	11	8

Leghorn	6	4½	5	4
Minorca (S.C. Black)	9	7½	7½	6½
New Hampshire	8½	6½	7½	5½
Orpington	10	8	8½	7
Plymouth Rock	9½	7½	8	6
Rhode Island Red	8½	6½	7½	5½
Sussex	9	7	7½	6
Wyandotte	8½	6½	7½	5½

*All the breeds listed lay brown-shelled eggs, except the Ancona, Leghorn, and Minorca. All these breeds have non-feathered shanks, except the Brahma.

Table 2.2: Type of Comb and Important Color Characteristics of Some Representative Breeds

Breeda	Type of comb	Color of ear-lobe	Color of skin	Color of shanks
Ancona	Single and rose	White	Yellow	Yellow
Australorp	Single	Red	White Yellow	Dark slate
Brahma (Light)	Pea	Red	Yellow	Yellow
Cornish (Dark)	Pea	Red	Yellow	Yellow
Delawares	Single	Red	Yellow	Yellow
Jersey Black Giant	Single	Red	Yellow	Black
Leghorn	Single and rose	White	White	Yellow
Minorca (S.C. Black)	Single	White	Yellow	Dark slate
New Hampshire	Single	Red	White	Yellow
Orpington (Buff and White)	Single	Red	Yellow	White
Plymouth Rock	Single	Red	Yellow	Yellow
Rhode Island Red	Single and rose	Red	White	Yellow
Sussex	Single	Red	Yellow	White
Wyandotte	Rose	Red		Yellow

* See footnote to Table 2.1.

RELATIVE POPULARITY OF BREEDS

In spite of the fact that there are so many different breeds and varieties, most of the purebred chickens kept in the United States belong to the following five breeds: Plymouth Rocks, Rhode Island Reds, New Hamp-shires, Wyandottes, and Leghorns. Delawares are increasing in numbers. There are no varieties of the New Hampshire breed, but among the other four breeds the following varieties are by far the most important: Barred Plymouth Rocks, White Plymouth Rocks, Single-comb Rhode Island Reds, White Wyandottes, and Single-comb White Leghorns. It is interesting to note that among these six varieties, three have white plumage, which presents a much simpler problem in breeding than is the case with most parti-colored breeds and varieties. Also, among the parti-colored breeds and varieties, it is easier to produce birds that meet approximate standard bred plumage requirements in Barred Plymouth Rocks, New Hampshires, Rhode Island Reds, and Delawares than in varieties having laced, penciled, and other complex plumage patterns.

White Leghorns are suitable primarily for market-egg production, and the other popular varieties, plus the New Hampshire breed, are kept primarily for egg and meat production. New Hampshires, White Plymouth Rocks, Barred Plymouth Rocks, and Delawares have been used extensively in broiler production.

3

GENERAL ANATOMY OF CHICKEN

Structurally birds share with mammals the distinction of being the most highly specialized of vertebrates. While basically being similar to mammals anatomically, evolution has brought about modifications for adoption to flight. The forelimb is changed to a wing in which the manus has been reduced by disappearance of digits and fusion of metacarpals.

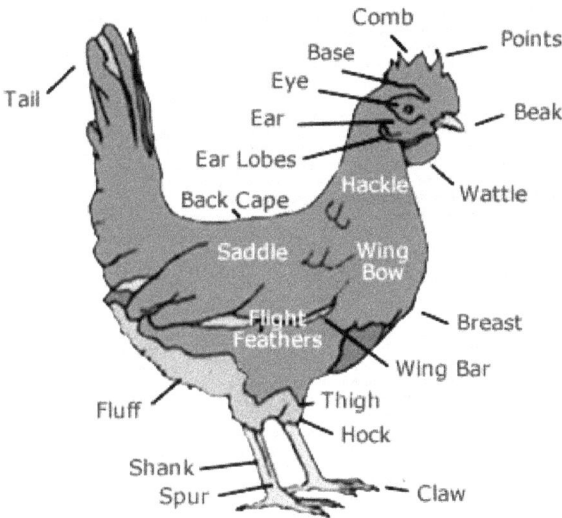

Fig. 3.1

Muscles of the pectoral region (breast), on the contrary are powerful to propel the bird in flight. The breast muscles are large and well developed. The magnitude of this development may be gathered from the fact that the breast muscles weight about as much as all the remaining muscles of the body together. They contribute one twelfth of the entire body weight of birds. The cervical, pectoral limb, pectoral girdle and pelvic limb muscles of birds are highly modified to meet the needs of locomotion.

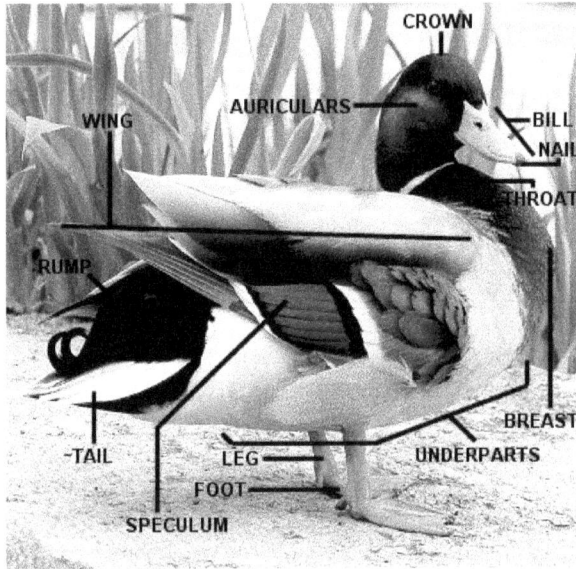

Fig. 3.2

Figure 3.1, 3.2, and 3.3 show the external anatomy of chicken, duck and turkey with names of various body parts:

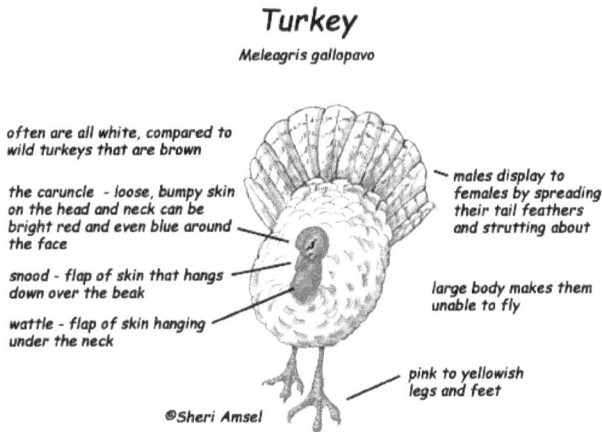

Fig. 3.3

Feathers of Fowl

The feathers are epidermal structure. They help to protect the birds from external injuries, keep body warm and help in flight. Feathers are arranged in rows within tract (pterylae) in the skin of poultry. The tracts are separated by non-feathered spaces (apteria).

Feathers can be divided in three types, (a) Plumules : are small downy feathers covered by contour feathers in adult birds. They provide insulation and help to retain body heat. (b) Filoplumes : are intermediate type of feathers, characterized by plumulaceous structure but having a distinct rhachis. They are hair like structures which remain after the bird has been plucked. (c) Contour feathers include all other feathers covering the body of bird e.g., flight feathers of wing and tail, the covert feathers which grow over the bases of the flight feathers and contour feathers which streamline the body. The parts of typical contour feathers are shaft; the lower part of the shaft is hallow and is called quill; at the joint of quill and shaft, there are fluffy filaments called quill; at the joint of quill and shaft, there are fluffy filaments called aftershaft; extending on either sides of the shaft are many parallel branches called barbs; the barbs in turn have branches known as barbules; the barbs in turn have branches known as barbules; the barbules have tiny hooks, the barbicels which serve to hold the parts of the feather solidly together.

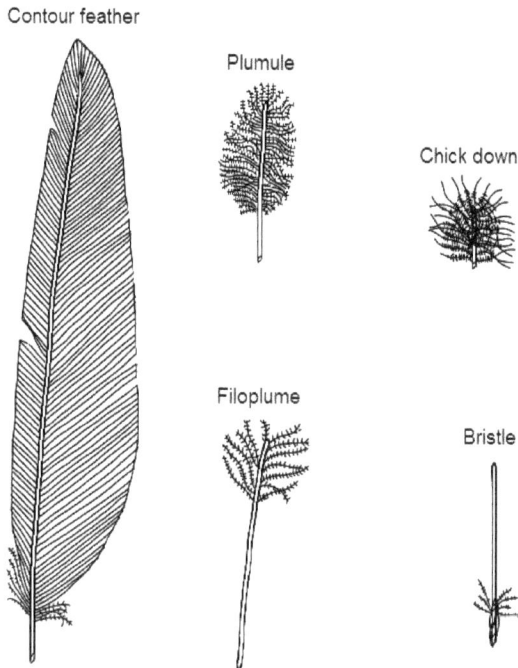

Contour feather

Plumule

Chick down

Filoplume

Bristle

Fig. 3.4

Skeleton System of Fowl

A view of the left half of the skeleton (Fig. 5) shows the skull, the thirteen cervical vertebrae of the neck, the seven thoracic vertebrae, the fused lumbosacral vertebra, the five or six coccygeal vertebrae of which the last produced by the union of several vertebrae and it is the largest. The latter vertebra is known as the pygostyl and forms the foundation for the feathers of the tail. The pelvis is formed by the union of ileum, ischium and pubis of the seven pairs of ribs. The first and second and sometimes the seventh do not reach the sternum. The phalanges are rudimentary while the metacarpus is in the form of a single bone produced by the union of three osseous elements corresponding to the first, second and third metacarpal bones of the mammalian limb. The ulna and radius form the bones of the forearm while stout and slightly curved humerus has an ovoid head for articulation with the scapula and coracoid. The clavicle is thin, rodlike and slightly bent.

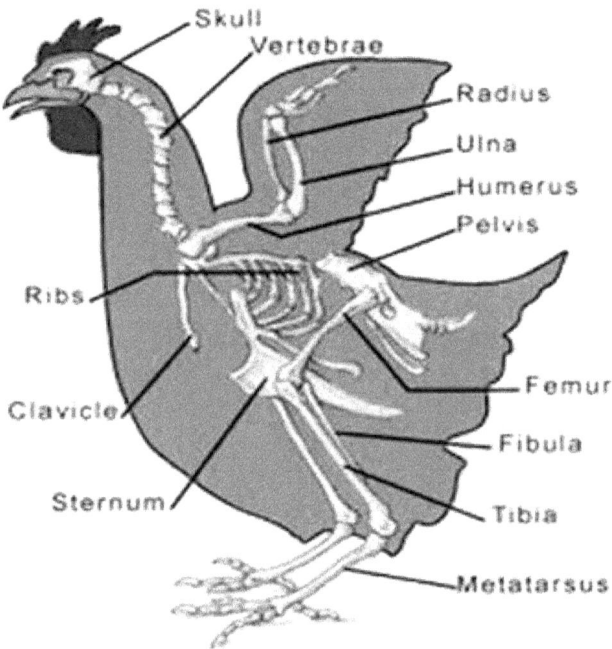

Fig. 3.5

The united clavicles form coming too close together during flight. The femur is stout and cylindrical. The tibia with its attached and poorly developed fibula is much longer than the femur. The adult metatarsus is represented by one long bone composed of second, third and fourth metatarsal bones in union. The phalangs form four digits.

The Respiratory System of Fowl

The nasal cavity is short and narrow while the trachea or windpipe is relatively long ending by branching into the right and left bronchi. The lungs are relatively small in comparison with the size of the thorax and are closely attached to the vertebrae and ribs. The axillary air sac is connected with the cranial end of the long transmitting air to the sternum, sternal ribs, shoulder-girdle and humerus. The anterior thoracic air sacs stretch from the clavicular to the abdominal sacs and unlike the other air sacs do not communicate with the interior of bones. The abdominal air sacs are large and communicate directly with the cavities of the sacrum, pelvis and femur.

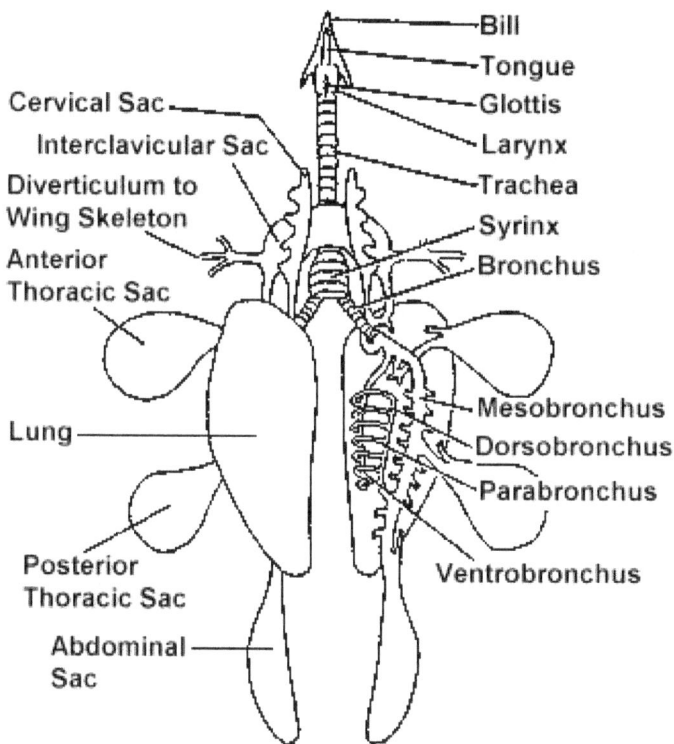

Fig. 3.6

The Digestive System of Fowl

The esophagus or gullet has at the thoracic inlet a marked dilation called crop. It serves to store food after rapid ingestion. The esophagus terminates at the glandular stomach or proventriculus which is relatively small but richly supplied with glands and lymphoid tissue. The muscular stomach or gizzard immediately succeeds the glandular stomach from which it is separated merely by a constriction. The gizzard is utilized for grinding feeds with the help of strong muscles and grits present in it. The small intestine beings at the exit from the gizzard and it is relatively of uniform caliber throughout its length. There are three parts of small intestine, namely duodenum, jejunum and ileum. Out of these only the first part can be distinguished easily. The elongated loop of the duodenum consisting of descending and the ascending limbs, extends as far posteriorly as the entrance to the pelvis. Between the limbs of the duodenum lies the pancreas. The ceca are blind tubes arising at the junction of the small and large intestine. The large intestine is very short, ending in the cloaca. Some anatomists describe the large intestine as consisting of two parts, the colon and rectum. The cloaca is the common opening for the digestive and urogential tracts. The large, dark brown liver is divided into two lobes, the right being the larger. The relatively large gall bladder lies on the right posterior part of the visceral surface of the liver.

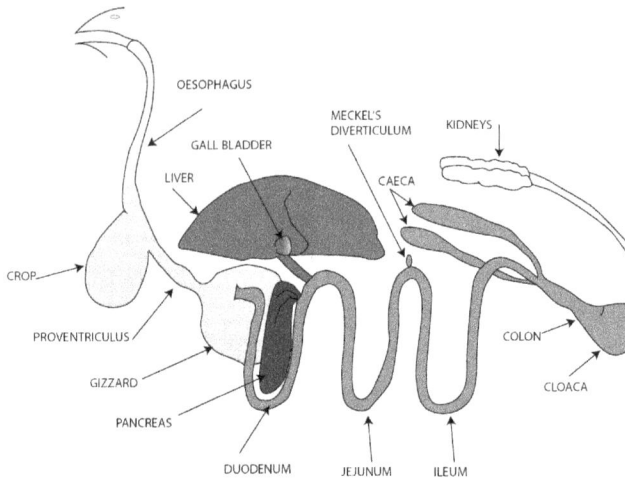

Fig. 3.7

The Reproductive System of Hen

The ovary with ova in various stages of development is an unpaired structure in the female birds (while there are two ovaries in the embryo, the right does not develop). The left ovary lies in the dorsal part of the abdominal cavity opposite the last two ribs. It weighs about 150 to 200 g. The oviduct varies in appearance according to its functional states; its anterior part corresponding to the fallopian tube of the mammal has a slit like opening leading called magnum and isthmus. Behind this the oviduct enlarges to form a wide thick walled tube which may be regarded as the homologous to mammalian uterus. The uterus is succeeded by vagina which opens into the cloaca at the left urethral opening.

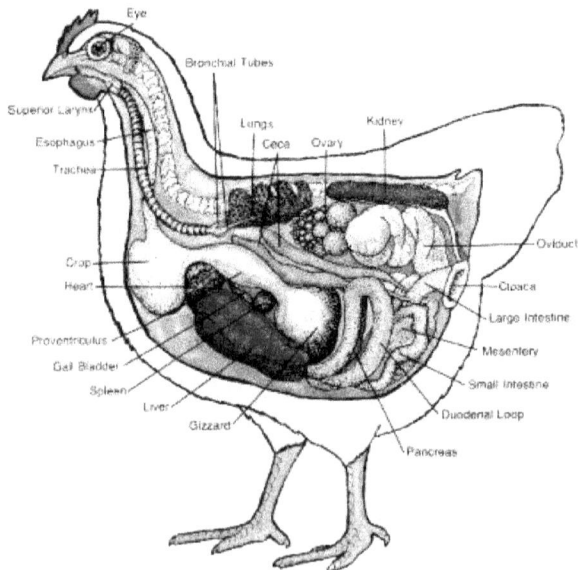

Fig. 3.8

The Endocrine System

There are two systems which help in coordination of different functions in animal body. The nervous system provides coordination by direct contact through nerves which carry massages from one organ to another. The second system is endocrine system. In this system chemical messenger or hormones are secreted by the endocrine or duct less glands which are carried through blood to the end organs where the actions are to be performed. Though this type of coordination is indirect but quite effective.

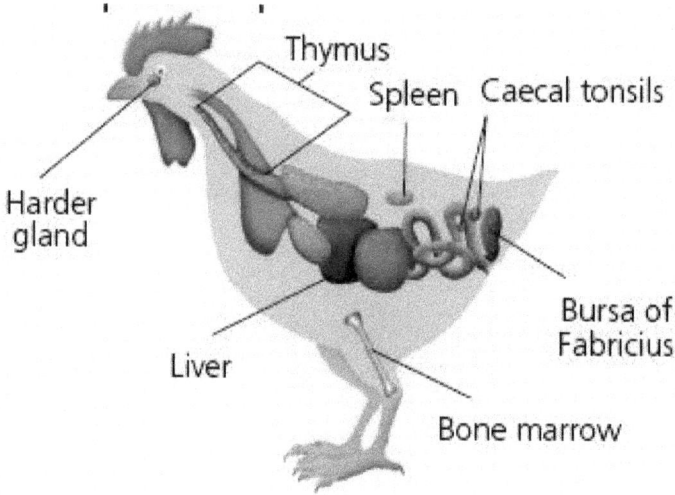

Fig. 3.9

The hormones may be defined as chemicals secreted in small amounts directly into the blood by glandular cells of endocrine glands. Although hormones circulate to all parts of the organism, but they stimulate or inhibit the rates of pre-existing reactions at the targets.

Approximate locations of different endocrine glands in chicken are shown in Fig. 10. The endocrine glands include ovary and tests (gonads), pituitary, thyroid, parathyroid, ultimobranchial body, adernal, pancreas, gastrointestinal tract. The pineal bodies and thymus which are sometime classified as endocrine glands are present in fowl, but their functions are still obscure. Anterior pituitary is considered as master endocrine gland as it regulates the secretion of other endocrine glands like of adrenal, thyroid and gonads. In turn, the anterior pituitary is mainly under the control of hypothalmus through different releasing factors.

4

POULTRY DISEASE AND THEIR CONTROL

The greatest threat to success of poultry enterprise is from disease. Serious illness is unlikely in a backyard flock, especially if you vaccinate the chickens. All the same, it's good to be aware of them in case you ever are wondering, is my chicken sick? Diseases can spread from wild birds and pests, so keep an eye out during your daily health checks for the symptoms listed below.

BACTERIAL DISEASES

- Escherichia Coli Infections
- Salmonelloses
- Paratyphoid Infections
- Fowl Cholera
- Riemerella Anatipestifer Infections
- Mycoplasma
- Necrotic Enteritis
- Cholangiohepatitis In Broiler Chickens
- Gangrenous Dermatitis
- Botulism
- Avian Tuberculosis

VIRAL DISEASES

- Viral Inclusion Body Hepatitis
- Haemorrhagic Enteritis Of Turkeys
- Egg Drop Syndrome -1976

- Adenovirus Group I - Associated Infections
- Infectious Bursal Disease (Gumboro)
- Infectious Bronchitis (Ib)
- Laryngotracheitis
- Swollen Head Syndrome
- Infectious Encephalomyelitis
- Newcastle Disease
- Fowl Pox
- Reovirus Infections

LARYNGOTRACHEITIS

- Swollen Head Syndrome
- Infectious Encephalomyelitis
- Newcastle Disease
- Fowl Pox
- Reovirus Infections

NEOPLASTIC DISEASES IN POULTRY

- Virus-Induced Neoplastic Diseases Marek's Disease
- Lymphoid Leukosis
- Myelocytomatosis
- Erythroblastosis
- Adenocarcinomatosis

PARASITIC DISEASES

- Coccidiosis
- Histomonosis
- Ascaridiosis
- Raillietinosis
- Knemidokoptosis

MYCOSES AND MYCOTOXICOSES

- Aspergillosis
- Aspergillus Granulomatous Dermatitis
- Aflatoxicosis
- Candidiasis
- Fusariotoxicoses

DEFICIENCY DISEASES

- vitamin B2 deficiency
- vitamin B1 deficiency
- vitamin E deficiency
- fatty liver haemorrhagic syndrome
- slipped tendon (perosis)

OTHER

- pulmonary hypertension (ascitis) syndrome in broiler chickens
- amyloidosis
- deep pectoral myopathy
- rupture of the gastrocnemius tendon in broiler breeders
- cage layer fatigue
- dyschondroplasia
- thyperkeratosis
- gout
- hyperandrogenism in broiler chickens
- effect of stickywilly (galium aparine) seeds on healthy status and production traits in broiler chickens
- gizzard impaction in turkey poults
- round heart in turkeys (dilated cardiomyopathy)
- acute selenium intoxication
- acute propane-butane intoxication
- spontaneous rupture of the caudial renal artery in turkeys
- subcutaneous emphysema
- gastrointestinal impaction
- Malformations

Poultry Disease and their Control

1. **Fowl-pox**

   Cause: It is caused by the virus.

   SYMPTOMS: The symptoms of this disease are of 3 types

   (i)   Cutaneous type: having scabs & pimples on comb, face and wattles: called dry pox.

   (ii) Diphtheritic type: in this type of symptoms mucus membraneusaffected in mouth and oesophagus.

   (iii) Infection of the nasal chambers with accompanying coryza like signs. Dry pox is more common.

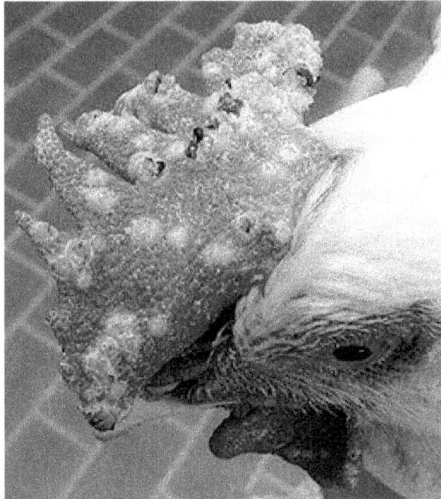

Fig: 4.1

Dry pox: In this disease the symptoms are comb, face, wattle are covered with scabs, pimples. Small white bumps on legs and feet which grow readily and turn yellow, later turn to dark brown lesions. After 2 to 3 weeks, the lesions dry up and become scaby.

Wet pox: Disease comprises loss of appetite, discharge from nostrils and accumulation of foamy material in the corner of eyes, dephtheric membrane in mouth, suffocation unless membrane removed, discharge from nose and face swelling, drop in egg production, mortality rate becomes 50 percent.

TREATMENT: There is no satisfactory treatment

TRANSMISSION: The diseases can transmited through scratches and wounds, virus carried by ectoparasites or mosquitoes.

Preventive Measures

1. Use good disinfection during outbreak
2. Spraying insecticide in and around premises
3. Stimulate appetite with wet mash or add antibiotic and vitamin mixture in drinking water.
4. Pigeon pox vaccine for laying birds (1/m)
5. Fowlpox "BM" strain at 14 to 15 weeks of age
6. Vaccination in growing period (4 to 5 weeks age) by fowl pox "BM" strain intramuscular (i/m)

2.   Marek' Disease (M.D.)

It is also known as – range paralysis; neural leucosis; skin leucosis. It is caused by the virus of herpes group VVMD.

SYMPTOMS: The disease affected birds will have some degree of paralysis, chickens in acute Form may not show this condition. Birds with paralysis unable to reach feed and water may die: acute form generally affects younger age group (6 to 10 wk.). Usually sudden death with high rate. In mature birds bilateral or unilateral paralysis of legs, wings or neck due to enlargement of various nerves inside the body. Other manifestation in this disease blindness and skin tumours are arises on the body.

TRANSMISSION: It is transmitted by way of air, saliva, nasal washings, feather follicles and droppings of infected birds.

PREVENTION

1. Attenuated virulent MD virus strains
2. Naturally occurring mild strains
3. Chickens blood containing mild MD agent but free from other agent
4. Herpes Turkey virus (HTV)

CONTROL

1. The birds should be maintained by strict isolation
2. Breeding stock resistant to MD

   AVIAN LEUCOSES COMPLEX (ALC): This is caused by filterable virus. its incubation period few weeks to 2 months.

   SYMPTOMS: Post martumlesions leions:

(i) **Neural type:** Sciatic trunk is enlargement & thickened Sciatic trunk

(ii) **Occular type:** Interior chamber of eye contains granular material, fading iris, irregular pupil, turbid exudate

(iii) **Visceral type:** spleen becomes enlarged which is greyish brown in colour, projecting greying tumours, enlarged liver, cauliflower like tumours on ovary, heart & kidney show similar lesions.

(iv) **In Osteoporosis:** Thickened long the bones becomes osteoporotic.

(v) **In Lymphomastosis:** paralysis of wings, legs or neck: In legs paralysis inward curving toes, moving difficult due to weakness.

TRANSMISSION: The disease can be transmitted by direct contact or through food, water or insect bite.

PREVENTION: Selective breeding, of restistant strain, hygeinic measures

TREATMENT: It should be treated by giving injection of potassium iodine. Tomato feeding suggested

4. Gumboro Disease or Ibd (Infectious Bursal Disease)

CAUSE: It is caused by the Ring serotype; highly contagious

TRANSMISSION: The disease can be transmited through contaminated litter, feed, and utensils and by the droppings of affected and litter mite are direct rectors.

SYMPTOMS: Diarrhea, depression, prostration and death. It cannot transmit by eggs (in chicks)

IN ADULT: White watery mucoid droppings, soiled vent feathers, loss of appetite; listlessness, less mortality but high morbidity.

PREVENTION & CONTROL

(1) Depopulation, destruction or distant removal of litter, thorough disinfection of equipment and houses.

(2) Avoid rearing layers and broiler chicken in – close vicinity

(3) Disinfect feet and hands of visitors,

(4) Incinerate dead birds; burn litter after removal

(5) Supplement low level vitamin

VACCINATION

(1) The chicks should be vaccinated at 5-7 days with LASOTA

(2) Give Gumbaro vaccination at 18-21 days and booster at 5-7 weeks.

5.   INFECTIOUS BRONCHITIS (I.B.)

CAUSE: IB is caused by virus

SYMPTOMS: The chicks causing this disease shows symptoms of Gasping, coughing, sneezing, discharges from eyes and nostrilis, egg production drops by 60 to 90%, egg quality deteriorates.

PREVENTION: It is prevented by:

(1) Vaccination with inactivated /attenuated live virus vaccine when day old with RD vaccine

(2) Vaccine is given through eye drop, nasal drop or aerosol spray or through drinking water.

CONTROL MEASURES:

(1) Proper sanitation

(2) Rearing birds of different ages separately

(3) Good management

6.   INFECTIOUS LARYNGOTRACHEITS (ILT)(AVIAN DIPTHERIA)

CAUSE: Through virus

SYMPTOMS: The chicks affected by this disease shows the symptoms: usually affects adults, respiratory distress, difficult breathing, coughing, blood coughed up, watery eyes, head & neck remain extended, break opens during each inhalation.

Transmission

(1) The Disease spreads rapidly bird to bird. Course about 2 to 4 weeks, mortality 5 to

7%.

(2) Aerosol method of transmission

(3) Contaminated litter, equipments, clothing, appliances

(4) Carrier birds after recovery from outbreak

PREVENTION: This can be presented by following measure:

(1) Stimulate feed consumption with wet mash, high level antibiotic feeds

(2) Vaccination

7. AVIAN ENCEPHATOMYLITIS

CAUSE: Entero-virus is responsible for this disease

TRANSMISSION: The disease can be transmitted through infected eggs, dropping of the birds and bird to bird direct contact.

NATURE: Mostly affected chicks are of age upto 6 weeks.

SYMPTOMS: The chicks suffering from this disease show inability to take food causing death. In coordination nervous signs, tremor of body, characterized by dullness depression, ataxia, sitting on haunches, inability to walk and paralysis, trembling head.

TREATMENT: The treatment of this disease are not effective

PREVENTION: It should be presented by following these parameters:

(1) Vaccination at 10 to 16 week age

(2) Purchase of birds from disease free stock

(3) Sanitation and hygienic measures

(4) Birds surviving attack be not used for breeding

(5) Cull the affected flock

8. INFECTIOUS VIRAL ARTHRITIS

CAUSE: Viral arthritis is caused by Reovirus

NATURE: It is generally affects meat type birds

SYMPTOMS: The birds shows the symptoms like lameness with swelling of hock joints, limited movement, swelling may be noted on foot pad and elbow joints.

TREATMENT: Not effective

CONTROL: Hygienic and sanitation measures

TRANSMISSION: It is transmitted by bird to bird contact, parent to offspring,, recovered birdsas carrier, because virus can persist for 250 days

9. AVIAN MONOCYSTOSIS

it is commonly known as blue comb, Pullet disease, X –disease

CAUSE: Virus,

TRANSMISSION: Unknown

SYMPTOMS: The birds suffering from this disease shows: dehydration, emaciation, fall in egg production, reduction in size of eggs, skin of legs become blue, depression, watery diarrhea.

TREATMENT: Not specific

CONTROL: These control measure should be followed

(1) Reduce dehydration by addition of molasses in water

(2) Adequate sanitation & hygienic measures

(3) Add vit. B complex in water

10. INFECTIOUS BODY HEPATITIS

CAUSE: It is caused through adenoviruses of DNA group

SYMPTOMS: The virus affects liver cells, ruffled feathers, dullness, emaciation, severe anaemia, heavy mortality.

TRANSMISSION: The virus can spread through directly from bird to bird, contamination by droppings and other secretion.

TREATMENT: Not specific

CONTROL: Spreading of disease can be controlled

(1) Proper disposal of affected birds

(2) Isolation of birds

(3) Adequate sanitation of the house and premises

BACTERIAL DISEASE

1. INFECTIOUS CORYZA (ROUP/INFECTIOUS CATARRH)

CAUSE: *Haemophilus paragallinarum*

SYMPTOMS: Bacteria cause the symptoms: discharge from eyes and nostrils, sneezing coughing, gasping, difficult breathing, swollen facial tissues and wattles

TRANSMISSION: It is transmitted by infected birds as carrier, free flying birds, contaminated food and water.

TREATMENT: The birds can be treated by the drug, Sulphaquinoxaline in feed and water, Sulphathiazole and streptomycin.

CONTROL MEASURES: The disease can be controlled by regular culling, good hygienic measures, birds from healthy stock, removal of carrier birds.

2. AVIAN COLI BACILLOSIS

CAUSED: By *Colisepticaemia, Escherichia coli*

TRANSMISSION: It is transmitted by insanitation & contamination of water and feed.

SYMPTOMS: The birds are suffering from swelling on joints, diarrhea of varying degree, wattle and comb, poor growth of young chicks, vulnerable to secondary infections, reduced production

CONTROL/PREVENTION: The birds can be presented by proper sanitation, reduce stress, proper ventilation, dry litter,

TREATMENT: Chicks are treated from medicine like Furazolidine, Furaltadone, Ampicillin, Chloramphenical, Oxytetracycline are more effective.

3. PULLORUM (BACILLARY WHITE DIARRHOEA; BWD)

CAUSED: By Salmonella pullorum

TRANSMISSION: The disease can be transmitted by egg, recovered birds as carrier contaminated food and water.

SYMPTOMS: Various type of symptoms are shown chicks after hatching die suddenly (50%), droppings of wings, general dejection, huddling together, brownish diarrhoea, great thirst, swelling of hock and foot joints, labored breathing, chalky white pasty faeces on vent region.

In adult: Dull, paleness of comb, depression, droppings of wing, weakness, lowered fertility, ruffled feathers.

CONTROL: It can be presented by good hygiene, routine agglutination test, culling of reactor, proper fumigation of incubator.

TREATMENT: Medicines of sulphamethoxasole group

(1) Sulphamezathine 16% (ICF) @30ml in 4 liters of water for 100 birds for 4 days

(2) Auromycin powder 8 to 16 gmper 10 litre of water

(3) Banif @ 1g per litre of water, Metaprim powder @ 12 gm per 10 litres of water for 5-7 days, Robatran granules @ 2gm. Per lit. of waterfor 7 days Mortin @ 1gm per litre of water for 7 days

(4) Furalatadone in drinking water @ 1.1 gm in 10 litres of water

4. FOWL TYPHOID (INFECTIOUS LEUKAEMIA)

CAUSE: It is very dreadful diseaseof fowl. It is caused by Salmonella gallinarum

TRANSMISSION: The birds contamination of food and water by droppings of infected bird, carrier birds, carcase, visitors and attendants feet, hands, clothes and shoes, ;through rats, dogs and cats as a mechanical transmission.

SYMPTOMS: The disease can be transmitted through dogs whenever the symptoms arises like yellow diarrhea, sudden death without appreciable manifestations, drooping of wings and tails, rapid breathing, rise in body temperature.

TREATMENT: Many drugs are popular test treating birds typhoid out drugs like, furazolidine, furaltadone, sulphodimidin, sulphamerazine. trimethoprinsulphadiazine/ sulphamethoxasole are affective. Chloromycetin group of medicine are good, other medicines like chloroplon, enterojat, pheniveting may also be used.

CONTROL: Good hygiene, culling of reactors after serological test, no entry of new bird without testing, live attenuated vaccine at 8 week of age.

5. FOWL PARATYPHOID

CAUSE: Just like human being birds also affected by Salmonella typhimurium, S. enteritides etc.

TRANSMISSION: Through infected breeding flocks, carrier birds, infected eggs, infected chicks after hatching, contaminated feed and water, rat, mice and insects, blood meal, meat meal, foot wears of visitors.

SYMPTOMS: Various symptoms are arises during these disease but some symptoms diarrhea pasting vents, somewhat similar to pullorum, birds huddle together, after drinking birds keel over backwards and die, closure of eye lids and dropping wings. Death rate max. 80%.

TREATMENT AND CONTROL: Some as fowl typhoid.

6. FOWL CHOLERA (AVIAN PASTEURELLOSIS)

CAUSE: It is caused by Pasteurellamultocda

SYMPTOMS: Greenish yellow diarrhea is sign of cholera found in nest, or roosts of dead birds, loss of appetite; sometime respiratory distress; increased thirst; swollen joints, comb and wattles; loss of weight; mortality up to 90% of affects birds.

TRANSMISSION: The cholera is spread very fast among birds by introduction of infected birds, contaminated feed and water by infected oral and nasal discharge, through subcutaneous wounds, conjunctiva, through hands and shoes of visitors; carrier birds after recovery may also spread disease.

TREATMENT: Hostacycline- 5gm in 4.5 litre water

Tetracycline- 5gm in 4.5 litre water

Should be given to the birds infected with cholera

CONTROL MEASURES: Removal of recovered carrier birds; introduction of new birds with removal of old flock; isolation of infected birds; keeping predators away from vicinity, minimize stress, proper sanitation.

7. AVIAN PSEUDOTUBERCULOSIS (YERSINIOSIS)

CAUSE: It is caused by bacteria Yersinia pseudotuberculosis

TRANSMISSION: The disease can transmitted through ingestion of infected feeds and water, infected soil through excretion of disease and dead birds, stress, malnutrition, through abraded skin, rodents.

SYMPTOMS: The birds infected from this disease shows symptoms like acute diarrhea/ septicaemia, dullness & depression, weakness ruffled feathers, distress breathing. Chronic form is characterized by somnolence stiff gait and discolouration of integument.

TREATMENT: Not effective

CONTROL: Same as fowl cholera.

5
POULTRY FARMING IN INDIA

Poultry Farming in India

Generally, poultry farming means, raising various types of domestic birds for the purpose of producing foods like eggs and meat. Nowadays, most of the people are using the poultry as the synonym of chickens. Because chickens are the widely raised poultry birds. Along with chickens ducks, geese, turkeys, guinea fowl, quails, peacock etc. are also popular domestic poultry birds. In India, various types of poultry birds are being raised from a long time ago. The largest number of poultry population in India is found in Andhra Pradesh followed by Tamil Nadu, Maharashtra, West Bengal, Karnataka, Bihar, Orissa, Kerala, Assam, Uttar Pradesh and Punjab. Some important urban areas like Mumbai, Pune, Nagpur, Kolkata, Delhi, Chandigarh, Bangalore, Chennai, Hyderabad, Shimla, Bhubaneswar, Ajmer etc. are raising poultry through a developed poultry farming systems. West Bengal and some other regions like Assam, Tamil Nadu, Kerala, Andhra Pradesh, Bihar, Orissa etc. are the most suitable place for duck farming. However, I am describing the benefits of commercial poultry farming in India and the steps for starting this business.

Benefits Of Poultry Farming In India

- There are many benefits of commercial poultry farming in India. The main benefits are listed below.
- Commercial poultry farming in India has created and still creating profitable business opportunity for the Entrepreneurs.
- Poultry farming business can provide a great employment source for the job seeking people.
- This is such a business in India that can never dry up.
- All types of poultry product has a great demand in the market inside India. And there are no religious taboo about consuming the poultry meat and eggs.

- Highly productive local and foreign breeds are available for commercial production.
- Required initial investment is not too high. You can start with small scale production and elaborate it gradually.
- Bank loans are available throughout the country.
- Numerous farms are available and you can easily learn about poultry farming from those established
- farmers.

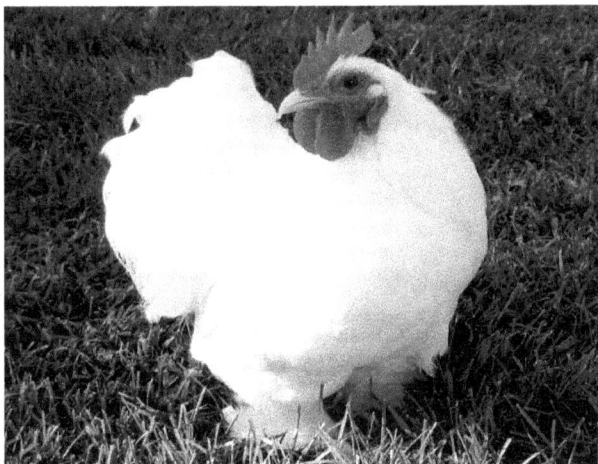

Fig: 5.1

Starting Commercial Poultry Farming in India

Starting commercial poultry farming business in India is not too easy. You have to go through some step by step process. To be successful in poultry farming in India, you have to go through the steps listed below.

CHOOSING SUITABLE LOCATION

The main and most important thing for poultry farming in India is selecting a suitable land. And it is the most expensive part of this business. For setting up commercial poultry production, it would be better if you have the land of your own. The area of the land depends on the number of birds you want to raise. Consider the following aspects while choosing land for commercial poultry farming business in India.

- Try to setup the farm in rural areas that is slightly far from the city. Because, land and labor are relatively cheaper in rural areas.
- Select a chaos and noise free calm and quiet place.
- The area of the land depends on the number of birds and farming system. Free range farming system requires more land than intensive system.
- The chosen area must have to have fresh and pollution free environment.

- Never setup the farm in rented land. Because, in rented land the land owner can force you to leave his land at anytime. So, it would be better if you are the owner of the land.

- While selecting land, ensure a great source of sufficient amount of fresh and clean water.

- The selected area must have to be free from all types of harmful animals and predators.

- Suitable transportation system is a must.

- Presence of a suitable market near the farm will be effective. You will be able to buy necessary commodities and sell your products easily in the market.

FARMING SYSTEM

For commercial poultry farming in India three systems are suitable according to the condition of India. And the suitable three systems are listed below.

1. Intensive System,

2. Semi-Intensive System and

3. Extensive System.

SELECTING BREEDS

Selecting high quality productive breeds is very important for successful poultry farming in India. There are numerous local and foreign high quality poultry breeds available in India. Choose proper breeds according to your desired production. If you want to start producing eggs commercially, select highly productive layer poultry breeds. For commercial meat production business, go with highly meat productive broiler poultry breeds. Contact with your nearest expert poultry producer to learn more about highly productive breeds. Common and mostly raised poultry breeds in India are of three types.

1. **Broilers:** The poultry breeds that is suitable for commercial meat production is known as broiler poultry. They are like meat producing machines. They consume foods and convert them to meat quickly. They grow fast and become suitable for slaughter purpose within very short time.

2. **Cockerels:** Cockerels are other types of meat producing poultry breeds. They also used for commercial meat production like broilers. But their growing rate is slower than broilers. They become hardy and can adopt themselves with the environment easily than the broilers. Cockerel meat is also very popular and has a great demand in India.

3. **Layers:** Various types of layer poultry are vary popular for commercial eggs production throughout the world. Some of them are very suitable for farming in India. Layers can be used for both commercial meat and egg production. There are some layer poultry breeds available which can lay upto 300 eggs per year.

Choose any of those breeds according to your desired production. While choosing breeds for commercial production, consider the availability of all types of necessary facilities. Visit your nearest local market and try to understand which product has a huge demand and price.

HOUSING/CAGE

Making a suitable poultry housing is another important factor for commercial production. But it is not too expensive like buying land. There are numerous ways for making a good house for the poultry birds. Always be sure that, the house or cage is sufficient and spacious enough to accommodate the birds with necessary space and facilities. In free range farming system, ensure sufficient amount of space for running and moving. The design of the house depends on the breeds and production type. However, while making a poultry house, consider the followings.

- Make a proper ventilation system in the house. Because, good ventilation system ensures good health and proper growth of the birds. So, the house must have to be well ventilated.

- Ensure flow of sufficient amount of fresh air and light inside the house.

- Try to make south faced house. This will help to entrance sufficient amount of clean and fresh air.

- If you go for large scale commercial production and make numerous house, then the distance from one house to another house will be at least 40 feet.

- Always keep the house clean and fresh. And clean it perfectly before bringing the chicks into the farm.

- Prevent all types of harmful animals and predators.

- Make good facilities so that rain water and cold wind can't enter inside the house.

- Try to build the house in a calm and quiet place.

- Make a suitable drainage system inside the house. It will help you to clean the house easily.

- Keep all equipment in proper distance inside the house. And always clean the house and equipment in a regular basis.

FEEDING

Feeding good quality and nutritious food keeps the poultry birds healthy and productive. So, good and high quality nutritious food is a must for commercial poultry production. There are numerous poultry feed producing companies available in India. They produce feeds for all types of poultry birds. You can easily use those food for your birds. If you want to prepare the feed at your home, then you must have to know the necessary nutrient elements in their food. And you also have to buy all those elements separately from the market and mix it in proper ratio. Along with providing fresh and nutritious food, always try to serve them sufficient amount of fresh and clean water according to their daily demands.

- Poultry feed
- Broiler poultry feed
- Layer poultry feed

CARE & MANAGEMENT

Always try to take good care of your birds. And good management ensure proper growth and production. The main threat of poultry farming in India is diseases. Thousands of farmer face huge loss due to various types of poultry diseases. So, always take good care of your birds and provide them nutritious food and clean water. Never try to mix contaminated or polluted food with their regular food. Vaccinate them timely and make a storage of some common and necessary medicines.

Marketing

The main benefits of poultry farming in India is easy marketing. You can easily sell your products in your nearest local market. So, you don't have to worry about marketing your products. If the local market located so far from your farm then transport the products very carefully

6

PRESENT STATUS OF INDIAN POULTRY

The present human population in the country is about 1210.19 million which is 17.5% of the world population and it is increasing in number by 1.9%. But the increase in crop productivity is only 1.7%. Though grains will remain the basic ingredients of world food supply, yet the demand for more animal protein will increase in future. There seems to be limited opportunities for increasing meat production (protein availability) from sheep, goat and beef cattle with existing slaughter rate and existing availability of fodder and pastures. The solution seems to remain with the poultry industry. Poultry is accepted universally as an economic converter of agricultural products and by products into a nutritionally balanced supplement fulfilling human requirements.

Poultry farming in India has registered a phenomenal growth during the past two and a half decades. From a gross annual value of production of less than Rs.40 crores in 1960, when commercial poultry farming first started it crossed Rs.1,000 crores in 1985 and Rs.1,400 crores in 1989 and 49,000 crores in 2011.

Today India ranks 3rd in world egg production and 5th largest poultry meat producer in the world. However, there is a large gap between the availability and requirements of poultry products. In light of ICMR recommendations against the requirements of 180 eggs and 11 kg poultry meat per person per year the present per capita availability is only 55 and 2.2 kg poultry meat per year by 2010 (FAO, USDA) which is far below the developed countries, leaving a big scope for further expansion by many folds.

The progress made in poultry industry has contributed significantly in improving in quality of nutrition available to millions of people. It is estimated that increasing consumption of one egg per year in India will create an additional 25,000 jobs. Over 6.5 million jobs are likely to be generated, if the target of 180 eggs and 11 kg of poultry meat per person per year is achieved.

The production of eggs, which was around 180 to 200 per bird per year has now reached an average range of 305 eggs for an improved layer. The broiler growth, which was considered as 1 kg, live weight in 8 weeks period has reached the stage of 1.75 kg per bird with 5-6 weeks. The growth of this industry during Seventh Five Year Plan has been envisaged at a very high rate.

Thus, through the concerted efforts of the Government of India and various other agencies, the poultry industry has grown tremendously. All these gains have been confined largely to the commercial sector and no significant increase in the egg and poultry output took place in the backyard sector. The initiative and vigour with which the private sector has come forward to popularize commercial poultry farming is encouraging. This tremendous growth in poultry sector has been possible mainly through the activity in the following areas.

(i) Development of high yielding layer and broiler breeds.

(ii) Improved health cover

(iii) Giving the poultry farmer the freedom to determine prices.

(iv) Increased awareness of the nutritive value of poultry products as well as enhanced purchasing power.

(v) Financing of Poultry Schemes.

(vi) Education and Training in Poultry Science in India.

(vii) Recent Advances in Poultry Nutrition.

(viii) Insurance of Poultry

(i) Development of high yielding layer and broiler breeds

Some notable achievements of the poultry breeding research undertaken in the country have been an evolution of a few commercial layers and broiler stocks which can be proud of and say are our own. Layers: These include ILI-80, HH-260, BH-78 and MY-Chix White egg layers released from Central Avian Research Institute (CARI) at Izatnagar; Central Poultry Breeding Farms (CPBF). Hessarghata and Bangalore and State Poultry Breeding Farm, Government of Karnataka respectively. Another tinted egg layer was also released from Central Poultry Breeding Farm, Bhubaneswar under the name Bhubaneswar Rhoda White.

At Venkateshwara Research and Breeding Farm, a joint venture with the ISA Breeders Inc. of the U.S., a new genetically superior layer breed was developed in early eighties. The Babcock breed produces upto 295 eggs a year at a lower feed consumption level than that of ordinary birds.

The Indian Council of Agricultural Research has evolved the following two improved layers.

(1) ILM-90 Hen housed egg production of more than 260 eggs upto 500 days of age with egg weight of more than 52 grams at 40 weeks of age.

(2) ILR-90 Hen housed egg production of above 245 eggs upto 500 days of age with more than 52 grams egg weight at 40 weeks of age. Some of the improved layers used presently are Starcross - 288; Starcross-579, BV300 etc.

Apart from these, Project Directorate on Poultry Hyderabad has developed two synthetic varieties named Vanaraja (dual purpose) and Gramapriya (layer) which can be reared in rural areas following backyard system.

Broilers: These include IBL-80, B-77, IBB-83, CA-42 and CH-47 commercial broilers released from Punjab Agricultural University, Ludhiana; CARI, Izatnagar; University of Agriculture Sciences, Bangalore and CPBF, Chandigarh respectively.

Another Venkateshwara Hatcheries Private Ltd. (VHPL) group company the Venco Research and Breeding Farm, a joint venture with Cobb Vantress Inc. of the U.S., developed and released the Ven Cobb broiler breed in early eighties.

Some of the improved broilers used presently are Hubbard, Anak-2000, Kasila, Caribro-91, Pearlbro-Samrat etc.

(ii) Improved health cover

As far as health cover is concerned, India has over 250 disease diagnostic laboratories and more than 20,000 veterinary hospitals. The facilities are mostly utilized for healthcare of large animals. The manpower in veterinary organisation is inadequately trained in poultry health care. The diagnostic facilities are also lacking in the hospitals. The supply of pharmaceuticals and biological products are satisfactory. Vaccine production in private sector is doing very well to meet the need and also export to various other countries.

(iii) Giving the poultry farmer the freedom to determine prices

Until the early Eighties, prices for eggs and poultry were dictated by traders and middlemen and were often un-remunerative. In 1981, egg prices crashed to such a level where 40 per cent of the farms were on the brink of closure.

If this situation has not been brought under control, the poultry sector would have stagnated at very low levels of production. The 1981 crisis resulted in the setting up of the National Egg Coordination Committee (NECC) originally by poultry farmers from four States with the intention of making the poultry farmer the arbiter in pricing. Over the years, NECC has been able to do just that prices of eggs are now fixed by the producers and are kept at levels that are remunerative to the producers and acceptable to consumers.

Still the eggs and meat marketing are handled by a few middleman and they control the market price without any regard to market economic forces. As a result, lion's share of profit is taken away and neither the producers nor the consumers are benefitted. The central Government through National Agricultural Cooperative Marketing Federation and the State Governments through Corporations and Boards are trying to interfere by providing price support to poultry farmers but so far no serious impact is seen. The government role to promote egg and meat marketing societies may be useful. Much needed attention is required towards the export of egg and meat in India, being at strategic position near the Middle East and Gulf countries, where there is a huge potential of export. To compete the international market, high quality, hygienic product at most competitive rates will be required. This scenario appears to be a long goal to achieve. A separate body from Agricultural Product Export Development authority

(APEDA) may be required to give full attention to promotion of eggs and meat and their products.

(iv) Increased awareness of the Nutritive value of eggs and Enhanced Purchasing Power

The increasing awareness of the nutritive value of eggs and thereby need for balance nutrition has led to changes in eating habits with vegetarians accepting eggs as part of their diet.

Simultaneously, there has been an increase in purchasing power, and more money is available for spending on quality food. With the changing food habits and increasing availability of eggs, there has been an increase in demand which is growing at about 10 per cent a year. Despite this, the egg industry experiences periodic slumps.

The key to the problem of slow growth is not per capita consumption, but per capita availability of eggs. Surveys conducted by the NECC in rural areas have shown that the demand for eggs and chicken is unfulfilled because they are not available in sufficient quantities, consequently, their prices are high. NECC is promoting egg consumption through television and other advertising media.

(v) Financing of Poultry Schemes

For the sake of supporting the full-fledged self sufficient poultry industry with complete sophistication in the fields of production, breeding stocks, high quality feeds, pharmaceuticals, medicines, poultry vaccines and equipments, the National Agricultural Bank and Rural Development (NABARD) along with National Commercial and Cooperative banks are financing a large number of poultry schemes all over the country for increasing production of eggs and broiler meat. This indicates the role that is being played by banking institutions in poultry development. The NABARD provides refinance assistance for poultry development for the following purposes:

1. Schemes for poultry breeding including financing of pure line poultry projects to produce grand parent stocks.

2. Financial assistance to hatcheries to produce commercial one day old broiler or layer chicks from poultry breeding stocks.

3. Financing for the setting up of commercial egg production farms of different sizes by small, medium and large farmers.

4. Financing for the setting up to commercial egg production farms of different sizes by small, medium and large commercial broiler farmers.

5. Financial assistance for the manufacture of poultry medicines and vaccines.

6. Financial assistance for egg marketing, broiler processing, preservation and marketing of poultry meat.

Apart from these, for small farmers there are several incentive schemes offered through District Rural Development Agencies (DRDA).

(vi) Education and Training of Poultry Science in India

There is well laid infrastructure for poultry education and training in the country. There are about 56 State Agricultural Universities (SAUs), many of them imparting graduate and post-graduate courses in poultry science. Besides the Central Avian Research

Institute (CARI); IPDA, Atwah, Surat, Gujarat, Institute of Poultry Management of India (IPMI) at Urulikanchan and Project Directorate on Poultry, Rajendranagar, Hyderabad are serving the purpose. The Central Poultry Development Organisations (CPDOs) located at four regions viz. Chandigarh, Bhubaneswar, Mumbai and Hasserghata have been playing a pivotal role in the implementation of the policies of the Government with respect to poultry. More specialised poultry training institutes for middle and lower levels are required.

(vii) Recent Advances in Poultry Nutrition

Nutrition is the science of the interaction of a nutrient with some part of a living organism. It is concerned with providing those elements of the external environment to the internal system of the birds which are essential to maintain the homeostatic conditions in them including maintenance of life, growth, egg production and resistance to diseases. The salient findings regarding recent advances in poultry nutrition are as follows:

1. Alternate Feed Resources

In the early sixties the priorities in poultry nutrition research were to eliminate from poultry ration feeds that man can use for himself. By the late seventies it is known that maize was not indispensible for poultry as energy source and that rice polishing, deoiled rice bran, tapioca, many kinds of millets, viz., jowar, bajra and ragi may be used as maize substitutes. Less damaged grain can replace 50% of the maize in poultry ration. Similarly the protein need may be met by judicious use of many oil seed meal other than conventional groundnut oil cakes, viz., sunflower oil meal, guar meal, mustard oil cakes, niger oil cake, cotton seed cake, karanja cake etc. Alternative to fish meal which is scarce and too expensive have also been found to be meat meal, meat-cum-bone-meal, liver residue meal etc.

2. Feed Processing

These findings helped to save maize and similar feeds from being used for poultry and feed costs were also considerably reduced. Haryana Agricultural University workers have attempted greater utilization of guar meal by appropriate ration modification while Punjab Agricultural University scientists have adopted fermentation technique for the same purpose. Using biotechnological approach the feeding value of guar meal, a by-product of guar gum industry has now been enhanced. Research has shown that deoiled sal seed meal could be used upto 5% in chick ration and upto 8% in layer diets as an energy source.

3. In-vitro Evaluation

Another area of considerable activity has been the development of in-vitro methodology for evaluation of feed ingredients and their protein quality. These methods employed the existence of correlation between the energy value of certain chemical identities in feed and the concentration of utilizable energy in the bird.

(*) ME = 432 + 27.91 (% C.P. + % EE x 2.25 + % available CHO)

(**) ME = 51.98 (% C.P. + % EE x 2.25 + % available carbohydrate)

(*) = Simple type of regression

(**) = Multiple type of regression

4. Nutrient Requirement

Scientists of the Poultry Research Division, IVRI; Punjab Agricultural University; Jawaharlal Nehru Krishi Viswavidyalaya, Jabalpur, Andhra Pradesh Agricultural University, Hyderabad are perhaps the leaders in this area. Based on the available information from the sources, specifications for some of the major nutrients in poultry rations have been developed by the BIS from time to time.

5. Limiting and Deleterious Factors

Considerable data are now available regarding some problematic feeding stuffs. In mustard oil cake, it is known that the presence of volatile isothiocynates and vinyl oxazolidienithone may limit the utilization of the cake to a great extent. The role of the various tannin components as well as of erucic acid may however be more important in inhibition of utilization of the cake by poultry. The different tannin fractions in the oil meals of Brassica species namely gallic acid, pyrogallol and pyrocatechol may not play a significant role in inhibiting the availability of the protein in the gut. On the other hand, Erucic acid - a major component of the fatty acid complement of mustard oil caused a significant depression in the body weight gain of chicks fed on the expeller mustard oil cake The toxicity due to erucic acid could be totally eliminated when the fatty acid was extracted from the cake.

Attempt has also been made to increase the level of guar meal (upto 20%) in poultry diet by enzymatic hydrolysis or fungal fermentation of the heimcellulosic gum components in the meal.

Tamil Nadu Veterinary & Animal Science University workers identified and quantified certain fatty acid fractions which inhibited the use of expeller rubber seed meal by poultry. Methods have been adopted to detoxify these factors for enhancing their use in birds.

Andhra Pradesh Agricultural University workers and also the workers of Bidhan Chandra Krishi Viswavidyalaya (BCKV) attempted to utilize the totally inedible Neem seed cake in poultry. The main neem seed toxin, azadirachtin, and others like melianloriol and salannin, all triterpenoid compounds are known to cause severe anti-feeding property either by a direct on palatability or by an indirect effect on the satiety centre in the brain. APAU worker has located a major portion of these toxic principles in the non-saponifiable fraction of the residual neem oil and employed -known chemical methods to totally detoxify the deleterious factor.

BCKV nutrition workers took the initiative not only to detoxify Karaja cake but also become successful in isolating some of the toxic principles and thereby made it possible for use of the processed deoiled cake throughout the country as livestock including poultry feed but with an exception of swine.

6. Mycotoxins in Feeds

Central Avian Research Institute and Jawaharlal Nehru Krishi Viswavidyalaya have contributed significantly to our knowledge on Aflatoxin. The tolerance level appear to be 0.5 ppm for broiler chicks beyond which growth depression, low feed intake and reduce feed efficiency were noticeable. The most effective methods are either autoclaving of infested material pretreated with a mixture of calcium hydroxide and formaldehyde or treatment with 5% ammonium solution.

7. Limitations

The essential component for fast and steady growth of poultry industry is production of economical balanced feed. At present, there are about 150 feed mills compounding about 30 million tons of feed of which about 1/3rd is consumed by birds. Except a few feed companies, most of them lack qualified staff, sufficient infrastructure and thus producing poor quality feed. There is no legislation to put the feed composition or proximate analysis on feed bags. As such poor quality and undesirable feed ingredients are commonly used for feed compounding. Added with this the feed testing laboratories are also inadequate where such feed could be got analysed at the time of poor performance. The shortage of good quality feed ingredients is currently the most serious hindrance in the progress of this industry and also in future, shortage of feed is likely to be a serious factor because poultry being the monogastric directly competes with human being for supply of cereal grains and other feed components.

Keeping in view the present rate of growth of poultry industry, feed requirement will increase in future. Nutritionists may have to look for more alternative sources of feed ingredients and this may also be the reason why most of research laboratories are involved in testing various non-conventional feeds like agricultural and industrial waste or by-products as feed.

(viii) Insurance of poultry

The scheme of poultry insurance has been first introduced in this country for the poultry farmers by the General Insurance Corporation (GIC) of India mainly to give financial security to investors of poultry. The policy covers loss against death of birds due to accident (including fire, lightening, flood, cyclone, famine, strike riot, etc.) or disease contracted or occurring during the period of insurance subject to some limitations. The details of these have been discussed in a chapter separately.

7

POULTRY MANAGEMENT

HOUSING MANAGEMENT

GENERAL LAYOUT OF POULTRY HOUSE

- Poultry house should be located away from residential and industrial area.
- It should have proper road facilities.
- It should have the basic amenities like water and electricity.
- Availability of farm labourers at relatively cheaper wages.
- Poultry house should be located in an elevated area and there should not be any water-logging.
- It should have proper ventilation.
- Layout should not allow visitors or outside vehicles near the sheds.
- The sheds should be so located that the fresh air first passes through the brooder shed, followed by grower and layer sheds. This will prevent the spread of diseases from layer houses to brooder house.
- There should be a minimum distance of 50-100 feet between chick and grower shed and the distance between grower and layer sheds should be of minimum 100 metre.
- The egg store room, office room and the feed store room should be located near entrance to minimize the movement of people around the poultry sheds.
- The disposal pit and sick room should be constructed only at the extreme end of the site.

DIFFERENT TYPES OF HOUSING FOR POULTRY

Deep Litter

- In this system the birds are kept in litter floor.
- Arrangement for feed, water and nest are made inside the house.
- Fresh litter materials spread on the floor.

- The birds are kept on suitable litter material of about 3" to 5" depth.
- Usually paddy husk, saw dust, ground nut hulls, chopped paddy straw or wood shavings are used as litter materials.
- This arrangement saves labour involved in frequent cleaning of faecal matter (droppings), however it needs periodical stirring.
- The litter is spread on the floor in layers of 2" height every fortnightly till the required drying is achieved.

Advantages

Vit B2 and Vit B12 are made available to birds from the litter material by the bacterial action.

- The welfare of birds is maintained to some extent.
- The deep litter manure is a useful fertilizer.
- Lesser nuisance from flies when compared to cage system.

Disadvantages

Because of the direct contact between bird and litter, bacterial and parasitic disease may be a problem.

Respiratory problems may emerge due to dust from the litter.

The cost of litter is an additional expenditure on production cost.

Faults in ventilation can have more serious consequences than in the cage system.

Cage System

This system involves rearing of poultry on raised wire netting floor in smaller compartments, called cages, either fitted with stands on floor of house or hanged from the roof.

It has been proved very efficient for laying operations, right from day-old to till disposal.

At present, 75% of commercial layers in the world are kept in cages.

Feeders and waterers are attached to cages from outside except nipple waterers, for which pipeline is installed through or above cages.

Auto-operated feeding trolleys and egg collection belts can also be used in this rearing system.

The droppings are either collected in trays underneath cages or on belts or on the floor or deep pit under cages, depending on type of cages.

Advantages

- Minimum floor space is needed.
- More number of eggs per hen can be received.
- Less feed wastage.
- Better feed efficiency.

- Protection from internal parasites and soil borne illnesses.
- Sick and unproductive birds can be easily identified and eliminated.
- Clean eggs production.
- Vices like egg eating, pecking is minimal.
- Broodiness is minimal.
- No need of litter material.
- Artificial Insemination (AI) can be adopted.

Disadvantages

- High initial investment cost.
- Handling of manure may be problem. Generally, flies become a greater nuisance.
- The incidence of blood spots in egg is more.

Problem of cage layer fatigue. (It is a condition, in which laying birds in cages develop lameness. It may be due to Ca and P deficiency but the exact reason is not known)

In case of broilers, incidence of breast blisters is more, especially when the broilers weight is more than 1.5 kg.

ELEVATED CAGE SYSTEM

- The height of the shed is raised by 6-7 feet using concrete pillars.
- The distance between two pillars is 10 feet.
- Two feet wide concrete platforms are made over the pillars. When 3 'M' type cages are arranged 4 platforms are needed.
- In case of 2 'M' and 2 'L' type cages are arranged 3 platforms are needed.
- When constructing platforms projecting angles or iron rods to be provided to fix the cages.
- The inter-platform distance is 6-7 feet depending upon the type of the cages used.
- The total height of the house is 20-25 feet and the width is 30-33 feet.
- This type of house provides sufficient ventilation in tropical countries.

CAGE REARING OF BROILERS

Broilers can also be reared on cages. Broiler cages are similar to that of grower cages. To prevent the breast blisters, the bottom of the cage may be coated with some plastic materials. The floor space requirement in cages is 50% of the floor space needed in deep-litter. The relative advantages and disadvantages of cage rearing of broilers are,

Advantages

- Higher density of rearing possible
- Easy to catch the birds at market time and hence reduces bruising
- No expenditure on litter

- No incidences of coccidiosis
- Reduced cannibalism
- Cleaning and disinfection easier
- Better growth and feed efficiency

Disadvantages

- Higher incidences of breast-blisters which increases carcass condemnations
- Higher incidences of crooked keel
- Wing bones will be more brittle which will be a disadvantage for the processor also.
- Birds are not having access to the unidentified growth factors in deep-litter system.
- Cleaning faecal-trays is not labour friendly.
- High initial investment on cages.
- Birds will be uncomfortable especially during summer.

POULTRY MANAGEMENT

Poultry management usually refers to the husbandry practices or production techniques that help to maximize the efficiency of production. Sound management practices are very essential to optimize production. Scientific poultry management aims at maximizing returns with minimum investment.

Brooder Management

Brooder house: Brooder house should be draft-free, rain-proof and protected against predators. Brooding pens should have windows with wire mesh for adequate ventilation. Too dusty environment irritates the respiratory tract of the chicks. Besides dust is one of the vehicles of transmission of diseases. Too much moisture causes ammonia fumes which irritate the respiratory tract and eyes. Good ventilation provides a comfortable environment without draft.

Sanitation and Hygiene

All movable equipments like feeders, waterers and hovers should be removed from the house, cleaned and disinfected. All litters are to be scraped and removed. The interior as well as exterior of the house should be cleaned under pressure. The house should be disinfected with any commercial disinfectant solution at the recommended concentration. Insecticide should be sprayed to avoid insect threat. Malathion spray/blow lamping or both can be used to control ticks and mites. New litter should be spread after each cleaning. The insecticides if necessary should be mixed with litter at recommended doses.

Litter

Suitable litter material like saw dust and paddy husk should be spread to a length of 5 cm depending upon their availability and cost. Mouldy material should not be used. The litter should be stirred at frequent intervals to prevent caking. Wet litters if any should be removed immediately and replaced by dry new litter. This prevents ammoniacal odour.

Brooding Temperature

Heating is very much essential to provide right temperature in the brooder house. Too high or too low a temperature slows down growth and causes mortality. During the first week the temperature should be 95°F (35°C) which may be reduced by 5°F per week during each successive week till 70°F (21•10C). The brooder should be switched on for at least 24 hours before the chicks arrive. As a rule of thumb the temperature inside the brooder house should be approximately 20°F (-6•7°C) below the brooder temperature Hanging of a maximum and minimum thermometer in each house is recommended to have a guide to control over the differences in the house temperature. The behavior of chicks provides better indication of whether they are getting the desired amount of heat. . When the temperature is less than required, the chicks try to get closer to the source of heat and huddle down under the brooder. When the temperature is too high, the chicks will get away from the source of heat and may even pant or gasp. When temperature is right, the chicks will be found evenly scattered. In hot weather, brooders are not necessary after the chicks are about 3 weeks old. Several devices can be used for providing artificial heat. Hover type electric brooders are by far the most common and practical these days. The temperature in these brooders is thermostatically controlled. Many a times the heat in the brooder house is provided by use of electric bulbs of different intensities. Regulation of temperature in such cases is difficult although not impossible. Infra¬red lamps are also very good for brooding. The height and number of infra-red lamps can be adjusted as per temperature requirement in the brooder house.

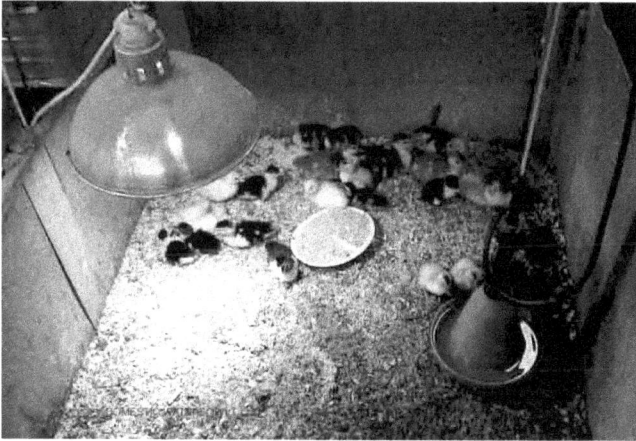

Brooder

Brooder Space

Brooder space of 7 to 10 sq inch (45-65 cm2) is recommended per chick. Thus a 1•80 m hover can hold 500 chicks When small pens are used for brooding, dimension of the house must be taken into consideration as overcrowding results in starve-outs, culls and increase in disease problems.

Brooder Guard

To prevent the straying of baby chicks from the source of heat, hover guards are placed 1•05 to 1•50 m from the edge of hover. Hover guard is not necessary after 1 week.

Floor Space

Floor space of 0.05 m^3 should be provided per chick to start with, which should be increased by 0.05 m^2 after every 4 weeks until the pullets are about 20 weeks of age. For broilers at least 0.1 m^2 of floor space for female chicks and 0.15 m^2 for male chicks should be provided till 8 weeks of age. Raising broiler pullets and cockerel chicks in the separate pens may be beneficial.

Water Space

Plentiful of clean and fresh water is very much essential. A provision of 50 linear cm of water space per 100 chicks for first two weeks has to be increased to 152-190 linear cm at 6 to 8 weeks. When changing from chick fountain to water trough the fountains are to be left in for several days till the chicks have located the new water source. Height of the waterers should be maintained at 2•5 cm above the back height of the chicks to reduce spoilage. Antibiotics or other stress medications may be added to water if desired. All waterers should be cleaned daily. It may be desirable to hold a few chicks one at a time and teach them to drink.

8

TERMS USES IN POULTRY PRODUCTION

A. I. = Artificial Insemination

Abdomen: Part of the body between vent end of the breast bone.

Abdominal Capacity: Distance between pelvic bones and end breast bone. This measurement is used for culling and selection of birds.

Abdominal dropsy: Swollen abdomen due to fluid in abdominal cavity usually common in over fat/old birds.

Acariasis: An infestation of animal with mites or ticks.

Acclimatization: Changes in physiology of birds when exposed to hanged environment.

Active immunity: It is natural immunity produced by administration of antigen derived from an infectious agent so that an animal mounts a specific immune response and achieves resistance to that agent.

Acute disease: When a disease appears rapidly it is called acute.

Additives are not essentially nutrients, but their presence increase nutritive value of diet, which may result in increased growth and egg production, increase in feed efficiency. They may be antibiotics, antioxidants, antifungals, vitamin supplements.

Addled egg: An egg in which embryo died between seventh and fourteenth day of incubation.

Adinovirus "EDS 76": The egg drop syndrome reported in 1976, is due to adino virus which has been designated 127, or BC14 causes depressed production together with loss in shell quality and colour (production of soft-shelled eggs or shell-less eggs).

Ad lib: Eating as much desired-means free of choice-under labour saving system poultry help themselves to eat ration as much as they wish.

Aflatoxin: A poisonous toxin produced by fungus Aspergillus flavus and found in groundnut cake and maize. It causes reduction in growth rate, poor egg production and immuno supression.

Agglutination: The process of causing germs to clump together.

AGMARK: Stands for "Agricultural Marketing". This label is given to agricultural and animal husbandry products which conforms to specific grade of quality and standards laid down.

Air Cell: Just newly egg laid has no air cell and has a temperature 105ºF, but when cools to room temperature, the liquid contents of egg contracts more than does the shell. Consequently inner shell membrane separates from outer to form the air cell. Later further increase in the size is due to evaporation of moisture from egg depending upon temperature, storage period, humidity, shell texture etc.

Air Puffs: After surgically caponisation air puffs sometimes appear which are incised to remove the air from under the skin.

Albumen: It is the egg white and makes 58% of egg weight. It is secreted in the magnum of oviduct. It is made up chiefly of 4 layers. The first layer is under the inner shell membrane called "Thin ablumen" which makes 21 percent of total white. It is followed by a thick layer which forms 55% of the egg white. Next to it is a "inner thin albumen" which is 17. 5% of total egg white and this is followed by a Chalaziferous of thick albumen which surrounds the yolk and forms about 6. 5% of total white.

Albumen index: It is the ratio obtained after dividing the height of the apparent dense albumen by average of its long and short diameters.

Alimentary tract: In poultry it consists of beak, tongue, gullet, oesophagus, crop, proventriculus, gizzard, small intestine, caeca, large intestine, cloaca and vent.

All mash feeding: One of the most preferred methods of feeding feed mixture in balanced form for all types of birds because birds cannot have opportunity of selective eating. It maybe fed in dry or wet form. All ingredients of feed are ground to optimum size and mixed with additives (flouring of any ingredient must be avoided).

Allantois: An organ of developing embryo which serves as embryonic respiratory organ, also absorbs albumen and calcium from shell.

American breeds: Under the classification American class includes Plymouth Rock, Wyndotte, Rhode Island Red, New Hampshire, Dominique Red and Java.

Ambient temperature: Surrounding temperature.

Ammonia: Reduce ventilation, crowding of birds, caking of litter, leaky waterers etc. causes high concentration of Ammonia in poultry house. Excess of Ammonia (more than 33 ppm) reduces growth of birds and egg production with respiratory disease and eye problems. Neutralise ammonia by adding superphosphate or phosphoric acid.

Ammiotic fluid: The watery fluid in which embryo floats within amnion.

An egg within egg: It is formed sometimes by reverse paristaltic action in which egg is forced back into funnel region of oviduct.

Roost: Perching place

R. O. P: Record of performance

Rose Comb: Broad solid comb flat on the top covered with small regular points with spike eg. wyandote

Roup: Name used to describe conditions affecting head and respiratory tract

Saddle: Rear part of back from from middle to base of tail.

Saddle Hanger: Long narrow lance shaped feather hanging down from the saddle of male fowl on both sides of body

Salmonella pullorum: BWD (bacillary White Diarrhoea)

Salseed meal: By product of sal fruit processing good source of energy and proteins but contains tannin hence has limited use in poultry diet

Salt Poisoning: Excess salt cause Poisoning symptom of lethargic, limb paralysis, difficult breathing

Saponins: Toxicant found in some feeds like Lucerne and soybean causes haemolysis of RBC

Scalder: A hot water tank thermostatically controlled used for dipping killed bids for easy removal of feathers

Scales: Horny tissue covering shank and feet

Scissor beak: Beak of bird having upper and lower mandible crossed.

Scratch feed: Granious part of ration

Scurf: Dandruff like scales on the comb

Secondries: Quill feather of wing which grow over the primaries and are visible when wings are closed.

Segmented worm: Tape worm

Salenium: Its requirement (0. 15 to 0. 2 ppm) depends upon vit E content in the feed . Fish meal is a good source of it.

Semen volume: In light breed cocks 0. 25 to 0. 5 ml and heavy breeds—0. 5 to 0. 75 ml.

Sesame seed meal: Can be used in poultry ration upto 50% of ground nut cake (GNC). It isdeficient in lysine but good source of methionine & tryptophane.

Sexing chicks: Chicks in hatcheries are sexed by cloacal identification, which consists of presence of rudimentary copulatry organ in males. This is called Japanese method. Breeders also use rate of feathering and colour pattern foq sexing day old chicks which are associated with sex linked gene.

Shank feathering: Is the characteristics of some breeds like Brahma, cochin etc.

Shank length: Can be used in growing period as an index to determine body weight.

Shape index: <u>Width of egg x 100</u>
　　　　　　Length of egg

Sheen: Lustrous and bright coloured plumage.

Shell strength: Can be measured by its thickness, resistance to puncturing or by shell weight per unit area.

Shell thickness: optimum 0. 3 mm

Shell: Make 11% of egg. It contains calcium carbonate 94% magnesium carbonate. 1% Calcium phosphate. 4% Organic matter . There are about 6000 to 8000 small pores on it for gaseous exchange of development embryo. It is covered with cuticle which is bacteriostatic in nature.

Shrinkage: It is loss in weight of bird from the time is picked up to the time delivered at processing plant. It depends upon distance of transit ration fed sex, temperature, humidity, etc.

Sib mating: Brother and sister mating (close mating)

Singeing: Removal of all hair without damaging skin.

Slips: Young male chicks chemically castrated(. tastes not removed). called slips

Slipped tendons: perosis

Slipped wing: a defect hangout when wings are closed

Social dominance: Dominant males in flocks mate more frequently than socially inferior one.

Spirochetosis: caused by Spirocheta gallinarum.

Stags: Male bird below ten month of age having tough meat called stags

Sternum: Breast bone

Stilbestrol: Used for chemical caponisation in cockerels@15mgm each .

Strains: Group of fowl within the variety.

Stress: Physiologically and mental tension

Stuck chicks: Shell sticking to chicks at hatching.

Stud mating: Hens are mating individually with male kept in coops.

Syndrome: A combination of symptoms resulting from single cause or so commonly occurring as to constitute a distinct clinical entity.

Tail covert: Curved feathers on the side of lower part of tail feather.

Tenderisation: A technique to convert tough meat of culled bird into soft andtender form by protolytic enzyme in combination with salts/ phosphate.

Thiamine: B1 deficiency symptoms are polyneuritis,nervous paralysis of legs,wings,and head

Ticks: Fowl ticks argas percious. it hide in cracks and crevices of house. Cause anorexia anaemia, weight loss reduced egg production and spirochaetosis.

Time switch: A swtch which puts light on automatically at set time.

Treading: Action of cock mating with hen.

Turning egg: This is done for hatching egg to prevent developing embryo from sticking to shell and also to allow distribution of heat . Turning of hatching eggis stopped on eighteen days of incubation.

Trypsin inhibitor: are the compounds capable of inhibiting protolytic activity of Trypsin and chemotrypsin. These are found in leguminous seed.

Ulcerative enteritis: Ulceration of small intestine is caused by clostridium colinum. Antibiotic treatment is effective.

Unsaturated fatty acids: Linoleic . linolenic and arachinodic.

Unsettable eggs: Cracked rotten mishappened,poor shell, double yolk tremulous air cell.

Vaccine: A suspension of killed or attenuated micro organism,when administered provides immunity.

Van wagner chart: This chart contains photographs of broken out eggs indicating quality . These are in used to determine quality by comparing the broken eggs.

Vent gleet: Known as cloacitis.

Vent pigmentation: When a pullet or hen is not laying the vent skin is yellow but when they are in in full lay get bleached showing pinkish white appearance so help in distinguishing a good layer from poor layer.

Vices: Are cannibalism, feather picking, toe pecking ,comb pecking , egg eating. etc.

Virus: Are ultramicroscopic organism,which can pass through chamberiand filter and multiplies only in living cells

Virulence: Competance of abnoxious agent to produce its effect.

Vermifuge: Substance which removed worms from intestine.

Vitality: A good physical and healthy conditions.

Walnut comb: Shaped like half walnut which is also a characteristics of Malay breed.

Water fowl: Breeds of duck and geese.

Waterers: Equipment should be such which keeps water clean cool and enough for birds.

Wet bulb thermometer: Apparatus to record degree of moisture present in the incubator ofegg chamber.

Wet mash systee: Poultry feed moistened and prepare withcrumbly state. It is wetted with water or butter milk. It prevents wasted of feed and increase efficiency but need more care.

Wheezing: Symptoms of respiratory disease and cold.

Whole grain feeding system: An old method of feeding in which several container containing separate grain are placed before bird to select and eat of theirchoice.

Wich egg: A very small egg with or without a minute yolk called cock egg and   witch eggs.

Wing bar: Bar of feathers across the mid of wing.

Wing bay: triangular part of folded wing between wig bar and wing point

Wing covert: Broad feather covering roots of secondary quill feathers.

W. P. S. A.   World Poultry Science Association

Wry tail: Tail carried permanently to one side.

Wry neck: Neck carried down to one side.

Yellow disease: Signs of disease black head, fowl pest.

9

POULTRY RELATED QUESTIONS

Questions and Answers on Poultry Management

Ques. 1: **How can the number of dirty eggs be reduced?**

Ans.   Clean nests, (do not allow hens to roost in nests), plenty of nests, (1 nest to 5 hens) clean, dry houses, clean graveled yards. Gather the eggs often

Ques. 2: **Do flocks do better confined or on range?**

Ans.   Breeding flocks generally do better on range and commercial egg flocks do better confined. It is difficult to use the same flock for both purposes.

Ques. 3: **Which are preferred for breeding, hens or pullets, and why?**

Ans.   Hens. (1) Hens have generally had a rest and hatchability is higher. (2) Hens have been culled and poor layers removed, (3) Hens lay larger eggs, producing larger, stronger chicks.

Ques. 4: **When should culling be done?**

Ans.   All the time throughout the year. Whenever a poor layer shows up, take her out.

Ques. 5: **What is the best way to break up broody hens?**

Ans.   Take them off the nest as soon as noticed, confine in a lighted, wire or slat bottomed coop, and feed them well.

Ques. 6: **When is the best time to select breeding stock?**

Ans.   Two years in advance. First, select large eggs of proper size, color and shape. Second, at two months of age select and mark largest, fastest growing cockerels and pullets. Third, cull closely at the beginning of the first laying season. Fourth, put into the breeding flock only those hens that have survived this rigid all year culling.

Ques. 7:   **How may naked back chickens be eliminated?**

Ans.   This is partially inherited, though crowding is partially responsible. In order to control it, remove all young stock showing any slow feathering characteristics. It may take several years to eliminate this trouble.

Ques. 8:   **What is the simplest way to control lice?**

Ans.   Nicotine sulfate put on the roost just before roosting time. (Directions for use printed on containers.) Sodium fluoride and blue ointment are also effective.

Ques. 9:   **What is a good spray for mites?**

Ans.   Any good wood preservative. (Obtained from lumber yards.)

Ques. 10:   **Why is it so important to remove males when the breeding season is over?**

Ans.   Male birds fertilize eggs and fertile eggs do not keep well. An infertile egg will not spoil nearly as rapidly as well fertile eggs.

Ques. 11:   **What is the difference between high quality hatching eggs and high quality market eggs?**

Ans.   None, except hatching eggs must be fertile and best market eggs must not. Select relatively short round eggs.

Ques. 12:   **How many feet of mash hopper space should be provided for 100 hens?**

Ans.   Twenty feet.

Ques. 13:   **When should Leghorns be hatched to make them the best ('a) breeders, (b) market egg producers?**

Ans.   February and March. These will molt and rest after three or four months of production. (b) April and May. These should lie through the winter.

Ques. 14:   **When should heavy breed hens behatched to. Make the best (a) breeders, (b) market stock?**

Ans. (a) As early as possible, February. (b) Same.

Ques. 15:   **How may one know whether production costs are high or low?**

Ans.   Keeping complete cost account records.

Ques. 16:   **Why are flocks of 50 or 500 hens recommended in Nebraska?**

Ans.   Eggs from small carelessly managed side-line flocks are usually inferior to the product of the larger commercial sized flock. Whenever a market surplus of any product fails to meet com- petition, it is usually at the mercy of the buyers. The cost of quality production from flocks under 500 is generally as much or more than can be realized from the sale of products. To reduce the cost, reduce the size of the flock to meet the home needs, or step it up to a size sufficient to justify labor saving equipment and efficient management in both production and marketing.

Ques. 17:   **What are the causes of unhealthy flocks?**

Ans.   Management, weak stock, late hatching, crowding, filth, incomplete rations, lack of feed, lack of feeder space, dirty or un- protected feeders and waterers.

Ques. 18:	**What is a good treatment for worms?**
Ans.	Try products of some reliable pharmaceutical company (ask your druggist for products of the firms making his drugs--prescription stock, not patent remedies.) Prevention through sanitation is easier, cheaper and more satisfactory. Any treatment to be effective must be followed with thorough sanitation.
Ques. 19:	**For what poultry diseases are vaccines recommended?**
Ans.	Thus far, chicken pox is the only poultry disease controlled through vaccination.
Ques. 20:	**Is blood testing for B. W. D. recommended? If so what method is used?**
Ans.	In hatchery breeding flocks, it is. In small farm flocks, it is doubtful. The quick method agglutination test using stained antigen is considered very satisfactory.
Ques. 21:	**What disinfectants are recommended for use about the poultry plant?**
Ans.	(a) Any of the phenol (carbolic acid) disinfectants may be used according to directions. (b) Chlorine disinfectants may be made from chlorinated lime. (Direct ions printed on containers. See Kansas Experiment Station Circular 130 on chlorine disinfectants.)
Ques. 22:	**How may soil be kept clean and free of disease producing organisms?**
Ans.	Sunshine, drainage, and cultivation will clean soil most satisfactorily.
Ques. 23:	**What are the chief items of cost in poultry keeping?**
Ans.	Feed, depreciation, replacement, interest on investment, and labor, with feed representing approximately on e-half of the total cost.
Ques. 24:	**What is the minimum cost of producing eggs from a flock of 100 hens laying (a) 60, (b) 50, (c) 40, (d) 30, and (e) 20 eggs a day? (Feed 'Costs of July, 1932 at three-fourths of a cent per pound.)**
Ans.	At 60, 50, 40, 30, and 20 eggs per day, the minimum cost per dozen should be about (a) 6% cents, (b) 8% cents, (c) 10% cents, (d) 13% cents, and (e) 20% cents.
Ques. 25:	**Which of the above letter classes include the average flocks of Nebraska?**
Ans.	Class "E".
Ques. 26:	**How may Nebraska hens be made more profitablc to the owners?**
Ans.	Through proper housing, feeding and management. (Keep production high and costs low.)
Ques. 27:	**How many more eggs would one need to obtain to justify an increase in the housing investment of from $1.50 per hen to $3.00 per hen?**
Ans.	At 15 cents per dozen f or eggs and 12% depreciation, it would require 15 more eggs per hen to cover this added cost.
Ques. 28:	**What kind of litter is recommended for laying hens? How much?**
Ans.	Generally whatever is available at lowest cost? Straw, hay, shavings, ground corn cobs, and sand have proved satisfactory. It is estimated that about one ton per

100 hens per year is sufficient.

Ques. 29: **How can chicks be marked so that their age and identity can be determined?**

Ans. By toe marks in the webs of the feet or numbered wing bands in the wings. Toe punching should be done at hatching time but wing banding may be done any time.

Ques. 30: **What is the average per cent of death loss of hens in Nebraska flocks?**

Ans. Cost account cooperators f or the last few years report about 12 per cent annual loss. Distributed in furtherance of cooperative agricultural extension work.Acts of May 8, 191 4, and June 30, 19 1 4. Extension Service of T h e University of Nebraska Agricultural College and U. S. Department of Agriculture cooperating. W. H. Brokaw, Director of Agricultural Extension Service.

Ques. 31: **What are the key animal hosts for animal reservoir viruses?**

Ans. Wild birds

Ques. 32: **The most important reservoir for highly pathogenic avian influenza H5N1 virus is?**

Ans. Domestic poultry

Ques. 33: **Which most accurately describes the purpose of surveillance in wild birds?**

Ans. Gain knowledge of the ecology and epidemiology of influenza in nature

Ques. 34: What is the main approach for doing surveillance for influenza A viruses in pigs?

Ans. Surveillance of animals with disease signs

Ques. 35: **What most accurately describes zoonotic infection risk?**

Ans. Sporadic infection occurs when humans are in close contact with animals

Ques. 36: **Which statement best describes surveillance for animals with influenza?**

Ans. Influenza surveillance in animals is intermittent around the globe and is more predominant in developed countries

Ques. 37: **Which of these methods is routinely used for confirming an influenza diagnosis?**

Ans. Culture and antigen identification

Ques. 38: **Haem agglutination inhibition measures which components of the immune response?**

Ans. Antibody response to Haemagglutinin